INTERACTIVE GROUP LEARNING

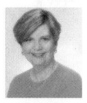

Deborah Ulrich, PhD, RN is an experienced nurse educator and national speaker who has been a prolific contributor to the nursing literature in the areas of group teaching strategies and cooperative learning. She has been teaching baccalaureate nursing and family studies courses for the past 25 years in university settings.

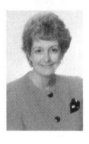

Kellie Glendon, MSN, RN,C is an experienced nurse educator certified in obstetrics. She has contributed much to the nursing literature in the areas of active student-centered learning and creative group-teaching techniques. She frequently speaks at national nurse educator conferences on innovative teaching in nursing curricula. She has been teaching associate-degree nursing students for the past 10 years.

INTERACTIVE GROUP LEARNING
STRATEGIES FOR NURSE EDUCATORS

Deborah L. Ulrich, PhD, RN
Kellie J. Glendon, MSN, RN, C

 SPRINGER PUBLISHING COMPANY

Springer Publishing Company, Inc.
536 Broadway
New York, NY 10012-3955

Cover design by Janet Joachim
Acquisitions Editor: Helvi Gold
Production Editor: Kathleen Kelly

99 00 01 02 03 / 5 4 3 2 1

Library of Congress Cataloging-in-Publication-Data

Ulrich, Deborah L.
    Interactive group learning : strategies for nurse educators / by
Deborah L. Ulrich and Kellie J. Glendon.
        p.   cm.
    Includes bibliographical references and index.
    ISBN 0-8261-1238-2
    1. Nursing—Study and teaching (Continuing education)   2. Social
groups.   I. Glendon, Kellie J.   II. Title.
    [DNLM: 1. Education. Nursing—methods.   2. Learning.
3. Group Structure.   WY 18U451 1999]
RT76.U46   1999
610.73'071'1—dc21
DNLM/DLC
for Library of Congress   98-31025
                                                                      CIP

Printed in the United States of America

Contents

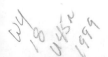

Preface

We decided to write this book because, as graduates of Miami University's Teaching Scholars Program, we had experienced the essence of teaching and learning and realized that teaching was more than telling. We began experimenting with group-learning strategies and found that students were capable of much more than we had been giving them credit for. They were asking thought-provoking questions and finding the answers themselves, as we facilitated this process.

As we have experimented with, published about, and spoken about these creative ways to teach, we have seen the interest and enthusiasm of other nursing faculty across the country. We want to share our insights and successes with them, so that they too can see their students develop intellectually.

DEBORAH ULRICH
KELLIE GLENDON

Acknowledgments

We wish to thank our students at Miami University who have helped us learn how to teach more effectively and how to empower them to become active lifelong learners.

We wish to thank Miami University's Alumni Teaching Scholars Program for bringing us together as colleagues and scholars interested in finding a better way to teach our students.

We also want to thank Joani Sheard for her encouragement and especially for her expertise in getting this book prepared for publication.

Introduction

It is certainly not current news that educators are beginning to look critically at the teaching learning process, yet it has been only in the last several years that nursing has begun to implement these new ideas. As veteran nurse educators, we have experimented with innovative and creative teaching strategies since the early 1990's, and we feel that we have gained much insight into the process of learning. We have discovered that a central tenet of effective learning is active involvement. Students who are actively involved in the learning process learn not only essential content more effectively, but also the crucial skills of communicating and interacting with others. More than ever before nurses are expected to think on their feet and efficiently apply their knowledge in situations with clients who are more acutely ill, are experiencing complex health problems, or present with a complicated and often dysfunctional family history. Nurses must be able to collaborate with other health care professionals, refer their clients to resources available in the community, as well as serve as an advocate for their clients and their families. These responsibilities require nurses to learn more than just necessary medical knowledge. It is essential for nurses to know how to work effectively with others, think critically, and communicate in speaking, writing, and interacting with others to benefit their clients. We have found that interactive group learning challenges students to meet these new learning essentials. This book is designed to help nurse educators or graduate students learning the art of teaching to implement this new group learning model in the undergraduate classroom and change the traditional education paradigm. It could also be used by staff educators for the continuing education of practicing nurses. These experienced nurses often bring a wealth of knowledge regarding real-life situations that augment the learning for the entire group.

This book is divided into seven chapters that present clear and practical ways to implement cooperative group learning methods. Examples can be quickly integrated into your existing teaching plan and will add the dimension of critical thinking and problem solving abilities, skills crucial for work in today's fast-changing health care environment.

Chapter 1 describes the shift in thinking about education from the traditional "Instruction Paradigm" to the new "Learning Paradigm." It details the advantages of this new paradigm and challenges you, the educator, to examine your curriculum and adapt your teaching methods to promote critical thinking and experiential learning through cooperative group techniques.

Chapter 2 presents our Comprehensive Group Learning Model designed to help you visualize the overall design of group learning through individual preparation, group interaction and sharing, and individual reflection. It explains the change in the teacher's role from one of information giver to one of facilitator and consultant, as well as the change of student role from one of passive recipient of knowledge to one of active participant in the learning process. This model allows you to plan a total class experience that requires not only group activities, but builds in individual accountability and preparation. The chapter concludes with an application of the total model in a strategy we call "Unfolding Cases and Unfolding Family Cases." These examples show you how this model can be implemented in its totality in a nursing classroom.

Chapter 3 discusses a multitude of cooperative learning strategies that can be used individually or in combination to cover the entire class content or as a break from traditional lecture. Each strategy is explained in enough detail to allow you, the teacher, to read it and immediately implement it in the classroom as a part of your already prepared lecture or class discussion. It also shows you how to combine a multitude of these cooperative strategies to teach an entire class, covering all of the content you need to teach. All of the strategies described stimulate group interaction and problem solving.

Chapter 4 introduces you to ways to involve students holistically through their senses. It will help you enhance their critical thinking abilities and allow them the experience of working with others all at the same time. This chapter shows you how to use drawings, photographs, videos, simulations, flow charts, and other media to help students learn the art of nursing.

Chapter 5 describes a variety of ways to help students learn factual information. Although we advocate teaching critical thinking and problem solving, students must first have general knowledge to use these higher-level thinking skills. This chapter details specific ways to help students prepare, prior to class, for group interaction. It also gives you numerous ideas for activities and games to help your students learn and remember information, as well as review for tests, licensure, or certification examinations.

Chapter 6 shows you how to use writing to increase learning and help students reflect on classroom content, readings, professional issues, and their own thinking. It discusses ways to use both group writing and individual writing assignments to increase insight and encourage perspective taking on the part of our students. This chapter enumerates the benefits of teaching students how to use writing as a method of communicating, critiquing others in a thoughtful and methodical way, and explaining their own thinking, to name a few.

Chapter 7 attempts to answer the common questions surrounding the use of groups in the nursing classroom. What do students think? How do faculty respond to this new learning paradigm? How can I make this change less uncomfortable for me? How does it change the way I grade individual students? These are but a few of the questions we will try to answer for you.

It is our hope that this handbook of interactive group learning strategies will assist you as you try to incorporate new ideas about teaching and learning into your classroom, as well as augment your existing repertoire of teaching strategies. We have found these strategies effective with all content common to general undergraduate nursing curricula, and think most any material could be covered using these methods. By reading this book, we hope to stimulate you to try new things by using our ideas, adapting our strategies to fit your own needs, or creating your own group learning techniques. Experiment! Have fun and share your new found enthusiasm with others—it's contagious and we all need to be revitalized as we continue to take on the important task of educating nurses for the next century.

CHAPTER 1

Changing Classroom Dynamics for the New Learning Paradigm

During the past decade, there has been a shift in thinking about the educational process among faculty in higher education. Historically, educators provided instruction, were the center of focus, and imparted their expertise to students in the form of a formal lecture. Barr and Tagg (1995, p. 13) coined this traditional teaching–learning structure the "Instruction Paradigm." It is based on the ideas of John Locke, who felt that a student's mind was a blank slate and that a teacher's job was to fill that slate. Hence, the idea of an active teacher and a passive student evolved and has remained the norm. The new structure of teaching–learning is referred to as the "Learning Paradigm" and emphasizes learning rather than teaching. It involves students actively constructing their own knowledge, whereas the teacher's job changes to one of manipulating the environment to allow active student *discovery* of knowledge (see Table 1.1). This philosophical shift in emphasis from teaching to learning demands that educators examine their curriculums and change their teaching methodologies to meet the new emphasis on critical thinking and problem solving.

No longer can faculty pour information into students and expect that this alone will prepare them for the needs of tomorrow's world (see Figure 1.1). Educators are beginning to consider critically the actual merits of this methodology of feeding students volumes of information much like a mother bird feeding her young. What could they expect to receive but the same information regurgitated back to them on an examination? Is this learning, or is it merely testing one's short-term memory? These are the questions that are now being contemplated by

1

TABLE 1.1   Comparison of Characteristics of the Old Instructional Paradigm Versus the New Learning Paradigm

Instructional Paradigm	Learning Paradigm
Teacher is the expert and center of knowledge	Teacher is the facilitator of learning
Individual and competitive learning	Group, cooperative, and collaborative learning
Students are passive in the learning process	Students are actively involved in the learning process
Teaching is "telling" and "giving" knowledge	Teaching is structuring the environment so that students "discover" knowledge
Students listen, record, memorize, and regurgitate information	Students apply knowledge, think critically, communicate effectively, and reflect on their own learning

educators worldwide as they look more deeply at the way we have traditionally viewed the teaching–learning process.

Although students do need to know certain facts before they can apply and critically think about them, memorization should not be the end of the learning process but the starting point. Bombarding students with new facts and information in lecture form and expecting them to apply the information in a clinical situation, sometimes the very next day, only overwhelms them (see Figure 1.2). They need time and help in learning to apply these essential facts after learning them cognitively. Learning experts report that students retain only 20% of what they hear in a lecture and even less of what they read on their own (Ekwall, 1976). In fact, Silberman (1996) notes that teachers speak 100 to 200 words per minute, but even a student who is concentrating can hear only 50 to 100 words per minute. However, more information is learned and retained when students are involved in the educational process and actually participate in the process (Dale, 1969). It appears that in using traditional methods, educators tend to ignore the processing of information and instead focus on presenting material. It is clear students retain more when they are active participants in processing the information rather than passive recipients of the knowledge (McKeachie, 1978). We also know that employers want to hire students who think critically, interact skillfully with others, and reflect on their own learning to improve themselves continuously. It is this kind of individual that will be successful now and in the next millennium, long after the facts they learned are outdated. So it is apparent that the

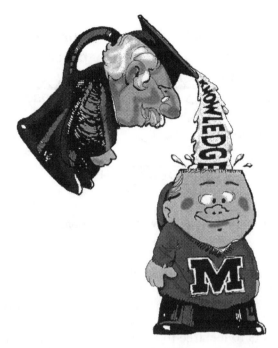

FIGURE 1.1   **Professor "pouring" knowledge into the student.**

outcomes faculty members need to produce in their students are the ability to think critically, problem solve, and remember and apply pertinent information—skills that will serve them well in life as well as in the role of a professional nurse.

CRITICAL THINKING AND REFLECTION

Critical thinking and reflection are two skills that we, as educators, need to require of our students. Thinking critically involves several skills that are best integrated through experiences (see Figure 1.3). An investigation of the literature related to critical thinking points out that there is substantial information, all defining, characterizing, and interpreting the term *critical thinking* in different but congruent ways. In reviewing the literature, Brookfield (1989) discovered that this concept has been likened to the development of logical reasoning, the use and testing of meaning, the application of reflective judgment, and the justification of beliefs. He sums it up best when he notes that critical thinking incorporates three closely related concepts: *emancipatory*

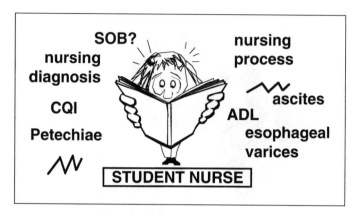

FIGURE 1.2   Bombarding students with information.

learning, dialectical thinking, and *reflective learning* (Brookfield, 1989, p. 12). *Emancipatory learning* refers to the individual being free from societal constraints that force them to conform to learning in only traditional styles where the professor is the center of knowledge. It requires students to feel free to brainstorm, think critically, and question authority without the fear of being "put down." *Dialectical thinking* assumes that change is a reality and, hence, promotes a constant process to discover truth. In other words, students need to be taught the only reality in life is change and that change is good and necessary for growth. This type of learning questions the norm and uses divergent thinking as a stimulus to further intellectual development. The *reflective* component of critical thinking involves looking at the justification for our beliefs and ideas or, more specifically, at the rationale for our actions. Why do I believe that, or what led me to this conclusion? If one is to accept something as truth, they must analyze the thought processes that brought them to acceptance of that fact.

Critical thinking in nursing similarly involves learning facts and applying them to common nursing situations. This involves examining multiple perspectives, analyzing and questioning assumptions, and interpreting information. Higher level thinking skills allow nurses to synthesize or reconstruct new concepts from data already known, as well as evaluate or judge the effectiveness of reasoned conclusions and their potential consequences. As practitioners, nurses will be faced with many decisions, some even life and death situations. Although there are certain facts nurses need to know to practice their profession safely, applying these facts to actual situations using the skill of critical thinking will enable them to solve problems effectively.

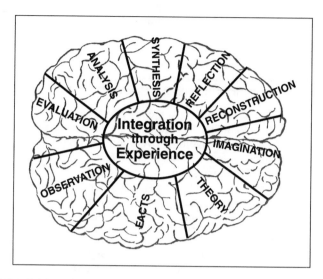

FIGURE 1.3   Critical thinking integrated through experience.

Faculty should feel obligated to teach students how to think and problem solve, not just teach realms of information. That conclusion implies there is a way in which to teach someone to think critically, and it is this ability that is necessary for faculty members to use as they go about their business of educating practitioners for the next century. This can be accomplished by devising teaching strategies that require critical thinking abilities, such as identifying similarities and differences, comparing multiple perspectives, interpreting and using theory, clarifying and analyzing issues, making interdisciplinary connections, and generating and assessing solutions (see Table 1.2). These can be actualized by involving students in group activities that require problem solving. One way faculty can stimulate student thinking through these activities is to include pertinent focused questions (Glendon & Ulrich, 1997) that direct student learning and help them concentrate on the most essential information and skills (see Table 1.3). These questions serve as a "map" to students as they learn to use these skills and practice applying them to the problems of nursing.

EXPERIENTIAL LEARNING

Experiential learning provides the link between critical thinking and student involvement. It is, in fact, the process we often use when

TABLE 1.2   Selection of Critical Thinking Abilities

Identification and recognition abilities
  Identifying and recognizing elements of reasoning
  Uncovering significant similarities and differences
  Recognizing contradictions, inconsistencies, and double standards

Comprehension abilities: comparing and clarifying
  Uncovering significant similarities and differences
  Refining generalizations and avoiding oversimplifications
  Clarifying and analyzing issues, conclusions, or beliefs
  Clarifying and analyzing the meanings of words or phrases
  Developing criteria for evaluation: clarifying values and standards
  Comparing and contrasting ideals with actual practice
  Reasoning dialogically: comparing perspectives, interpretations, or theories

Application abilities
  Comparing analogous situations: transferring insights to new contexts
  Clarifying and analyzing the meanings of words or phrases
  Analyzing and evaluating arguments, interpretations, beliefs, or theories
  Analyzing and evaluating actions or policies
  Rethinking your thinking: metacognition
  Exploring thoughts underlying feelings and feelings underlying thoughts

Synthesis abilities
  Reasoning dialogically: comparing perspectives, interpretations, or theories
  Comparing analogous situations: transferring insights to new contexts
  Making interdisciplinary connections
  Reasoning dialectically: evaluating perspectives, interpretations, or theories

Evaluation abilities
  Refining generalizations and avoiding oversimplifications
  Comparing and contrasting ideals with actual practice
  Designing and carrying out tests of concepts, theories, and hypotheses
  Analyzing and evaluating arguments, interpretations, beliefs, or theories
  Analyzing and evaluating actions or policies
  Rethinking your thinking: metacognition
  Exploring thoughts underlying feelings and feelings underlying thoughts
  Reasoning dialectically: evaluating perspectives, interpretations, or theories
  Evaluating the credibility of sources of information
  Generating and assessing solutions
  Questioning deeply: raising and pursuing root or significant questions

Abilities to create or generate
  Designing and carrying out tests of concepts, theories, and hypotheses
  Generating and assessing solutions
  Creating concepts, arguments, or theories

From Paul, R. (1993). *Critical thinking: How to prepare students for a rapidly changing world.* Santa Rosa, CA: Foundation for Critical Thinking. Reprinted by permission.

TABLE 1.3   Examples of Focused Questions

What could be happening in each of the following scenarios?
What data support your assumption/conclusion?
What data are needed to help clarify the situation?
What information did you use from your previous knowledge to reach
the decision?
What effect would this have?
What (other things) _____ would be important to assess
(e.g., lab data)?
Describe/explain _____.
What immediate actions need to be planned?
What resources need to be used?
What alternatives are there?
Explain the rationale supporting your conclusions.
How did you feel about your choice?
What were the benefits/disadvantages of a certain course of action?
What were the consequences of your action?
What teaching strategies would you use?
Create an argument for or against _____.
How would you coordinate _____?

From Glendon, K., & Ulrich, D. (1997). Unfolding cases: An experiential learning model. *Nurse Educator, 22,* 15–18. Reprinted with permission.

teaching the skill of critical thinking. Dewey (1944) observed, as early as 1915, that learning occurs in society as a result of social interaction. He thought that formal education needed to be active and that students needed to be involved, or experience the knowledge firsthand, if they were to discover the "connections of things" (Dewey, 1944, p. 340). The Gestalt theorists Wetheimer and later Koffka, Kohler, and Lewin studied the relationship or link between experience (as defined by Dewey) and learning (Bigge, 1971). They determined that experiential learning helped students develop reflective thinking skills that, in turn, enabled them to transfer knowledge to new situations (Bigge, 1971). Many educators have used the principles of Dewey and the Gestalt theorists to develop teaching strategies, such as simulations, role play, and laboratory experiences. Frederick (1990) used stories, writing exercises, music, and dynamic visuals to "connect" the student's life experiences to the subject matter at hand. By tapping the student holistically (i.e., physically, intellectually, emotionally, and spiritually), students are more actively involved or connected to the learning experience. They, in fact, experience learning firsthand as they are forced to participate actively in the process. Experiential learning activities that tap the senses and the emotional and psychological facets of the student extend the effectiveness of the learning outcome produced.

COOPERATIVE LEARNING

Cooperative learning adds yet another dimension to Fredericks's ideas (1990), the social dimension, which binds students together to solve problems or learn specific content. It is the process by which students implement the teacher-planned activities. "Cooperative learning is an interactive teaching strategy that stimulates critical thinking, fosters a feeling of community within the group and promotes individual responsibility for learning through group process techniques" (Glendon & Ulrich, 1992a, p. 37). Students learn not only how to think and analyze but also how to work effectively in teams, learning outcomes useful in the work world.

Group processing through cooperative structures involves students working in groups of four to six members. Groups can be formed by random choices, self-selection, or teacher decisions. Working in heterogeneous groups gives students experiences in interacting with others that come from multiple perspectives, such as different cultures, achievement levels, learning styles, sex, and ages. Hence, deliberately formed groups that are heterogeneous seem to work best. Group work helps them develop crucial communication skills needed for building consensus, disagreeing with others with divergent ideas while maintaining respect for one another, encouraging and including others in discussion, and resolving conflict. In fact, cooperative learning stresses the development of social skills as well as cognitive ones.

Cooperative learning is not a new concept in education. In fact, much research has been done dealing with the effectiveness of these methods. Research has consistently shown that cooperative learning methods not only produce greater academic achievement than do traditional methods of instruction but also improve student self-esteem, promote positive attitudes about school, and encourage interaction between students of different types (Sharan, 1980; Slavin, 1980; Slavin, 1983a, 1983b). Although, traditionally, most research has been conducted on the kindergarten through 12th-grade level, one early college-level nursing study found that African-American nursing students studying cooperatively achieved higher scores on state board examinations than a control group that studied independently (Frierson, 1986). In recent years, both interest in and research on cooperative learning has consistently increased in higher education and the same benefits as seen at younger educational levels have been found (Cooper & Mueck,

1990; Johnson, Johnson, & Smith, 1991; Qin, Johnson, & Johnson, 1995). In fact, research has shown that "cooperative efforts produce higher quality problem solving than do competitive efforts on a wide variety of problems that require different cognitive processes to solve" (Qin et al., 1995, p. 139). In summary, there seems to be four major benefits of cooperative learning: (a) increased student involvement, (b) enhancement of critical thinking, (c) improved communication, and (d) promotion of responsibility for learning.

Although the terms *group learning* and *cooperative learning* are often used synonymously, they have substantial differences. Cooperative learning has several characteristics that distinguish it from traditional small-group learning, group projects, or buzz groups (Cuseo, 1992). Cooperative-learning groups are intentionally formed to assure heterogeneity; they do not form by chance or student choice. Generally these groups meet regularly for an extended period of time and do not change every class period as small-group work groups may. This longevity promotes cohesiveness and a group bond. Efforts are aimed, through specific activities, to promote cooperation and interdependence among team members. Team-building activities, individual rewards as incentives for group cooperation, and team roles are examples of such activities that are commonplace in cooperative groups. Individual and group accountability is present in cooperative groups. The group is responsible for meeting defined goals, and each individual is responsible for doing his or her fair share to realize that group goal. Each person has an identifiable contribution to the group's success. The use of a peer evaluation form (see Table 1.4) ensures that group members' evaluations of other group members is considered in each individual's grade.

Communication and social interaction skills are stressed as groups interact, and specific exercises are included in the group work assignments to assure this focus. In cooperative learning groups, the instructor acts as a facilitator and consultant as the group processes their task, whereas in traditional group work the instructor leaves the students to go about their work with little structure.

Kagan (1989–1990, p. 38) illustrates the point that all classroom instruction has a particular structure, even the "whole class question-and-answer" strategy, but the level of participation of each student— and, hence, learning—is in question in this and other traditional structures. For example, in this structure, the teacher calls on one student, and the student tries to answer correctly. With the "whole class question and answer," it is usually higher achieving students that have the most poise, confidence, and knowledge level that participate, whereas lower achievers with less self-esteem may sit and listen, or even tune out. Learning is more apt to be meaningful if all students take part in

TABLE 1.4   Peer Evaluation

Evaluate each member in your group, excluding yourself. In any case, when you give a 1 or 5, you must explain your reasoning in the comment section.

1 = Never; 2 = Rarely; 3 = Sometimes; 4 = Usually; 5 = Always

	Group Members:				
	1	2	3	4	5
1. I was satisfied with the quality of their work.					
2. I was satisfied with the quantity of their work.					
3. They attended all group meetings.					
4. They did their share of the work and contributed equally.					
5. They showed respect for all group members and used good group-processing skills.					

Totals

Comments:

the group-learning structures. These structures designed by the authors and other cooperative-learning experts tend to multiply the learning potential in the classroom by assuring that more than a select few students are involved. Examples of these structures applied to nursing education and staff development are provided in detail throughout the book. In addition, there are several cooperative learning workbooks that are excellent references for college teachers wanting to change their teaching style to include group learning structures (Cooper, Prescott, Cook, Smith, Mueck, & Cuseo, 1990; Goodsell, Maber, & Tinto, 1992; Johnson, Johnson, & Smith, 1991; Kagan, 1992).

In summary, the new learning paradigm is here, and it is time for nurse educators to analyze its value and experiment with it in their own classrooms. Together we can improve the learning, skill, and potential of the professional nurses of tomorrow.

CHAPTER 2

Experiential Comprehensive Group-Learning Model

I t is readily apparent that to teach in this new learning paradigm, faculty members need to mesh the concepts of critical thinking, experiential learning, and reflection in such a way to accomplish the desired educational outcomes of producing students who can think, analyze, problem solve, communicate, and evaluate their own effectiveness to assure self-improvement. However, facts and knowledge cannot be forgotten as they are prerequisite to one's ability to analyze and problem solve. How can we, as faculty, assure that our students receive both? Figure 2.1 describes the use of a *Comprehensive Group-Learning Model* that does just that. Faculty can use it to design individual classes or even entire courses that meet the desired outcomes of learning facts as well as critical analyses.

In this model, the teacher's role changes to one of facilitator and consultant. The facilitator acts as a guide by creating an environment that is conducive to learning. After the teacher sets up the experience, the students first prepare individually out of class through teacher-constructed study guides, worksheets, and other exercises that require them to attain essential factual information, and then, in groups, become active participants in solving the problem or completing the task at hand. The problem often includes focused questions (see Table 1.3) that guide students to practice and apply the principles of critical thinking. These problem-based activities are processed through cooperative-learning strategies or structures that enhance or augment the level of participation of every student. Through teacher-planned activities, student groups generate solutions and share their results with the

11

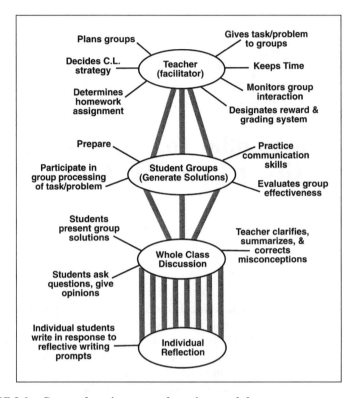

FIGURE 2.1   Comprehensive group learning model.

entire class. The facilitator (teacher) circulates in the room, keeping time, clarifying the task, and monitoring the groups' interactions. Students are encouraged by the facilitator to promote cohesiveness of their groups by practicing social relationship skills and communication techniques, such as active listening, paraphrasing, clarifying, brainstorming, and conflict resolution. The teacher than facilitates a total class interaction, promoting a higher level of discussion and analysis, which highlights the critical thinking component. Students are finally asked to reflect on their own learning experiences through a short writing exercise. This writing exercise provides closure to the discussion, adds a new component for thought, or encourages students to evaluate their own effectiveness. Table 2.1 lists some selected reflective writing prompts. Although reflective writing provides an individual critical thinking moment, it is essential to the overall goals of learning, helping students to improve themselves continuously by encouraging them to think about what they have learned and how it

TABLE 2.1   Reflective-Thinking and Writing Prompts for Writing Exercises

What are your beliefs about _____?

How have your beliefs about _____ been changed?

What is your interpretation of _____?

Write a reaction to _____ from the perspective of the nurse/patient/family.

Write a critique of your group's discussion.

List two ways in which your group could be more effective.

Describe one way to keep a group member from dominating the discussion.

Describe one way to help a shy group member to contribute to the discussion.

Summarize the essence of the argument for or against _____.

Write supporting statements of an argument that you truly do not support.

Write objectives for your future learning needs.

Considering your participation in the group today, list three ways you can improve your effectiveness in communicating your ideas, getting others to listen, explaining your viewpoint, or leading your group.

Ask a question on the current topic—a variation that causes the student to ponder another aspect.

From Glendon, K., & Ulrich, D. (1997). Unfolding cases: An experiential learning model. *Nurse Educator, 22,* 15–18. Reprinted with permission.

will personally affect them. It is an important element completing the Comprehensive Group-Learning Model.

Although most of this book gives detailed examples of specific group-learning strategies, or focuses on selected aspects of the whole model, the following *Unfolding Cases* and *Unfolding Family Cases* examples demonstrate the use of this comprehensive group-learning model in its totality. Although the authors recommend using the entire model, faculty can also use pieces or parts of it independently. Application of the total model as an overview will be presented first, with ideas on how to use selected parts of the model detailed in later chapters. This learning model can be used as the basis for a class or course, depending on the instructor's objectives.

UNFOLDING CASES (Glendon & Ulrich, 1997)

Educators today are realizing the value of designing strategies that actively involve students for outcomes of the new learning paradigm. Nurse educators in particular are aware of the need to prepare student nurses for managing clients with various needs in an environment driven by demands of cost containment and managed care plans. The reality is that data are often complicated and continually changing as clients' health status improves or declines and as information is obtained from other health care providers, clients, and their families. Rarely does the nurse know the whole picture before care. With shortened hospital stays, the nurse must obtain, analyze, and synthesize available data about the patient and plan nursing care accordingly. This requires an experienced level of critical thinking and communicating. Our Unfolding Cases (Glendon & Ulrich, 1997) design meets the goal of actively involving students as well as allowing them practice time to individually, as well as collectively, solve problems they may encounter in clinical situations. The net effect is a greater repertoire of skills and perspectives to apply when faced with new problems and challenges.

As described by Glendon and Ulrich (1997), Unfolding Cases is a variation and extension of the frequently used strategy of case studies (Dailey, 1992). It presents an ever-changing case or scenario that students process sequentially. An Unfolding Case usually contains three paragraphs, although individual educators could design as many additional paragraphs as they need to meet their learning goals. The first paragraph sets the stage for the scenario. It includes pertinent background information related to the characters of the case, the initial situation they find themselves in, and focused questions. Groups of students interact to process the focused questions and then share their interactions with the entire class. To facilitate discussion and interaction among peers, cooperative-learning strategies, such as *Roundtable* (Kagan, 1992), *Think-Pair-Share* (Lyman, 1987), and *Pass the Problem* (Kagan, 1992), are used (Glendon & Ulrich, 1992a). Detailed specific instruction for these cooperative-learning strategies are included in Chapter 3. Then, the second paragraph is revealed. This paragraph could reflect a change in time, build on the last paragraph, or include a new focus. Students again process the questions of this paragraph and share the findings through cooperative-learning exercises. At this point, any further paragraphs are sequentially revealed, building on the case, or changing its focus. The final step is an individual reflective writing exercise that could encourage students to plan for their future learning needs, to think about and share individual reactions, or to reflect on and thus deepen the learning experience.

In building the structure of the case, the professor needs to address seven specific areas: purpose of the case, biographical data, context, content, focused questions, cooperative-learning strategies, and reflective writing. In the *purpose of the case* professors must first clarify the intent of this exercise, or what it is they want the students to gain from participating in the case. Is this case to be used for one entire class, a series of classes, or as a post–clinical wrap-up session? What are the expected outcomes? Is it to teach content or apply previously learned concepts? Professors need to plan expected answers to augment discussion when needed and to ensure all pertinent information is discussed.

The case example in Table 2.2 was designed with many purposes in mind. One of the purposes was to allow students the opportunity to apply assessment findings to the pathophysiology of heart defects. The given set of data indicated some of the classic signs of cardiac disease in children, which included low weight, history of respiratory illness, and clinical signs of dyspnea on exertion, fatigue, cyanosis, and clubbing of the fingers. The professor would expect students to investigate further clinical signs, such as oxygen saturation, respiratory rate, need for oxygen, adventitious lung sounds, heart murmur, heart rate and rhythm, peripheral pulses, capillary refill, peripheral edema, and hematocrit. Students are challenged to apply knowledge of data given as well as data missing, and the professor must be prepared to clarify and add to the discussion.

Biographical data on all characters of the case need to be created. Information, such as age, sex, culture, socioeconomic status, and educational level, needs to be included. Such information brings the case to life, highlighting the individuality of the client situation. In this specific case, a 10-year-old white child, her mother, and a nurse are identified. Paragraph one of the case includes information one might find in a chart or kardex as well as some assessment data obtained from the night nurse (see Table 2.2).

Context refers to several different aspects, such as environment, historical information, resources available, or the situation at hand. Context could also refer to biographical information, such as a person's gender, cultural perspective, or one's frame of reference. The content of the case example occurs in the hospital, beginning with admission data and moving to planning for discharge. The example case highlights the situation the nurse is faced with when bleeding occurs post–cardiac catheterization (see Table 2.2).

Content includes a variety of concepts, such as pathophysiology, treatments, medications, health promotion and prevention concepts, legal and ethical issues, laboratory findings, teaching, and discharge planning as seen in the example case study (see Table 2.2). These concepts represent the knowledge that students must be able to apply in clinical situations and are often the focus of the questions asked of the student groups.

Focused questions are used to encourage students to brainstorm and problem solve the issues inherent in the case. These questions are designed to stimulate critical thinking related to the nurse educator's learning outcomes. Typical questions might direct students to evaluate

TABLE 2.2   Case Example for Nursing Education

Learning Outcomes

After processing the case, the student will be able to
- Apply assessment findings to pathophysiology of heart defects.
- Apply principles of preoperative and postoperative nursing care for a cardiac catheterization.
- Plan individualized discharge teaching for the client/family.
- Use resources for identified problems.

Paragraph 1

Day 1, 0800: Molly is a 10-year-old Caucasian girl admitted to Children's Hospital with cardiomyopathy. She has been seen several times in recent years for pneumonia. A cardiac catheterization is planned for tomorrow. Her weight is 27.7 kg. The night nurse indicates in report that Molly has dyspnea on exertion and tires easily. She also has circumoral cyanosis and clubbing of the fingers.

Focused Questions and Cooperative-Learning Strategies

Group 1	Relate the current clinical data to child's diagnosis. What data are important to collect considering the child's diagnosis and symptoms? What would you expect to find?	**Roundtable**
Group 2	What standardized teaching is included in preoperative and postoperative preparation for a cardiac catheterization? How would you individualize this teaching for a 10-year-old child?	**Roundtable**
Group 3	Develop and prioritize a list of nursing diagnoses for Molly followed by three nursing interventions for each diagnosis.	**Roundtable**

After all three groups have finished, each group must pass the problem to another group. Each group processes a new list of nursing diagnoses and interventions, refining and adding more to the list; groups report their findings.

Paragraph 2

Day 2, 0930, cardiac catheterization: The child returns from the procedure. Her color remains dusky around the lips. RR18, no retracting of nasal flaring noted. Bp WNL. R femoral site has dressing saturated with bright red blood. Peripheral pulses are strong and equal.

(continued)

16

TABLE 2.2   (Continued)

Focused Questions and Cooperative Learning Strategies

Pairs of students	What could be happening with the introduction of this new data? What data are needed to support your conclusion? What do you do if you decide there are abnormalities?	**Think-Pair-Share** Pairs are called on to report.

Paragraph 3

Discharge day: Instructions are written as follows: Home O_2 therapy at night. Protimes once per week. Medications of digoxin 0.125 mg q12 hours po and captopril 12.5 mg po q8 hours. You already called the company that supplies home O_2 therapy and find the family has been denied service because of a lack of insurance. You find out mom is not on welfare. In your interactions with mom yesterday, she confides to you that she has a "nervous" problem and takes numerous medications that cost a lot of money. Mom also needs frequent reminding related to the child's needs, and you are beginning to wonder if she is capable of following a medication schedule for Molly.

Focused Questions and Cooperative-Learning Strategies

Groups 1–3	Considering your role as coordinator of care, how would you plan for discharge? What course of action is indicated with the addition of new data related to mom? Consider the options and decide on the best approach.	**Roundtable. Report each group's findings.**

Reflective-Writing Prompt

Suppose that when you reported excessive bleeding to the physician after the cardiac catheterization, the physician responded with, "lots of kids bleed, don't worry about it." How would you feel, and what would you do?

From Glendon, K., & Ulrich, D. (1997). Unfolding cases: An experiential learning model. *Nurse Educator, 22,* 15–18. Reprinted with permission.

information given in the case, or it may require them to anticipate expected findings from their previous knowledge (Browne & Keeley, 1990) (see Table 1.3). In the case example, students were asked to apply knowledge of pathophysiology to plan appropriate nursing interventions for Molly. It may even ask students to identify pros and cons of an intervention or course of action. Students in the case explore what to do about bleeding post–cardiac catheterization (see Table 2.2).

Strategies used in processing the case are based on cooperative learning principles. A key benefit of cooperative learning is that it encourages students to communicate with their peers. The ability to articulate their ideas is enhanced in this interactive process. Students realize that having to explain a concept to someone else ensures understanding and enhances their own memory. Some strategies that work well include *Think-Pair-Share* (Lyman, 1987), *Roundtable* (Kagan, 1992), and *Pass the Problem* (Kagan, 1992), to name a few, although additional cooperative strategies could be used (Ulrich & Glendon, 1994, 1995). Chapter 3 gives detailed step-by-step instructions and examples of these techniques. Because the professor assigns each student group a separate question to process, groups work individually on their tasks and ultimately share results with the entire class. As students stand and report their group's ideas, confidence is gained in communicating with others, yet another benefit of the exercise.

Reflective writing is used to complete the entire exercise. It serves as a method of encouraging individual student reflection on the learning that has occurred, gives students something further to think about related to the current topic, or encourages self-reflection of strengths and areas needing improvement. Writing exercises need be only a paragraph or two in length and require only minutes of time to complete (Cross & Angelo, 1988). In the case example (Table 2.2), students are asked to respond by reacting individually to a physician's inappropriate comment, "lots of kids bleed, don't worry about it." This reflective prompt stems from the focused question in paragraph 2 (see Table 2.2), when the student is asked: "What course of action is indicated if an abnormal finding occurs?" The logical answer is to apply pressure to prevent hemorrhage and call the physician to report the finding. The added dimension of an inappropriate physician response stimulates the student to consider individually the options, actions, and consequences with yet another dilemma complicating the situation.

As in the first Unfolding Case example, Table 2.3 highlights another specific physiological problem that can be covered using an interactive format. The five paragraphs of this case follow Kerry, a spinal cord–injured client, from the scene of the accident to the emergency room through hospitalization and rehabilitation. Through the use of cooperative-learning strategies, groups of students process focused questions related to the desired learning outcomes expected by the faculty member (see Table 2.3). The reflective-writing prompt changes the focus of the case from one of dealing with physiological data to the emotional components.

Table 2.4 gives another Unfolding Case example dealing with a chemically dependent peer. Staff development educators as well as nurse educators could use this case for their staff or students to process solutions to this common problem. This three-paragraph case requires participants to examine issues related to this situation before actually experiencing it. It is hoped that this exercise will stimulate discussion related to the proper procedures that need to be followed for

TABLE 2.3   Unfolding Case Example Including Possible Answers With a Spinal Cord Injury Scenario

Learning Outcomes
1. List priorities of care at the scene of the accident.
2. List the main cause of respiratory distress in the spinal cord–injured patient.
3. Recognize appropriate interventions as the client changes over the course of injury and rehabilitation.
4. Verbalize potential or actual nursing problems related to the data in the case.
5. Recognize signs of impending collaborative problems and intervene appropriately.

Paragraph 1
Kerry Fisher, 19-year-old college sophomore, is involved in a head-on collision. At the scene of the accident, you find Kerry sitting in the front driver's seat. You note the windshield is broken in a large star pattern directly over the steering wheel. Kerry is unconscious.

Focused Questions and Cooperative-Learning Strategies

What would your priorities be?   **Roundtable**

Possible answers:
1. Assess and establish an airway if needed using jaw-thrust; assess for bleeding/circulation problems.
2. Immobilize head/neck; do not move him—potential for spinal cord injury.
3. Assess for other injuries—head or internal injury.

Paragraph 2
Kerry develops shallow breathing with periods of apnea en route to the hospital. The hospital is 3 minutes away, and the rescue team decided to administer oxygen with an Ambu bag.

Focused Questions and Cooperative-Learning Strategies

What is the main cause of respiratory distress in a spinal   **Think-Pair-Share**
   cord–injured patient?

Possible answer:
Spinal shock.

Paragraph 3
On admission to the ER, BP is 80/40, p 42, R12, T 95, bowel sounds are absent, and bladder is distended. He is unconscious, and breathing is irregular.

Focused Questions and Cooperative-Learning Strategies

What interventions do you anticipate?   **Roundtable/Pass the Problem**

Possible answers:
Assess and manage respiratory distress; ABGs, intubate, O_2, Swanz and cardiac monitoring; vasopressors for BP and p; NG tube, Foley catheter, methyprednisolone (Medrol) for cord edema; x-rays, MRI, later EMG to assess level of injury.

(continued)

19

TABLE 2.3   Unfolding Case Example Including Possible Answers With a Spinal Cord Injury Scenario *(Continued)*

Paragraph 4

Kerry is past the spinal shock, and neurogenic response is under control. His spine is stabilized with cervical traction, and he is placed on a Stryker frame. An initial home visit to assess Kerry's access to his home reveals several concrete stairs to all entrances. His mother indicates that there are no available funds to construct a ramp.

Focused Questions and Cooperative-Learning Strategies

What nursing problems do you anticipate as healing occurs?   **Think-Pair-Share**

Possible answers:
1. Impaired physical mobility (skin-turn, pin care, massage bony prominences-decubiti)
2. Impaired gas exchange/ineffective breathing patterns—level of injury will impede breathing; need help with cough; deep breathing; suctioning—limit as bradycardia
3. Elimination—self-cath, reflex voiding; suppository/timing
4. Sexual dysfunction
5. Self-esteem
6. Potential infection (pins, UTI, URI)
7. Potential impaired skin integrity (decubiti)
8. Impaired home maintenance; lack of finances to construct home for wheelchair

Paragraph 5

Kerry's Foley catheter was removed 6 hours ago. When you assessed him 30 minutes ago, he was lying in bed talking to his parents. VS, p 96, 120/60, R20, T98.3. Kerry complained of a severe pounding headache. You repeat his VS and find p50, 180/110, R28, T98.5. You notice goose bumps on his arms.

Focused Questions and Cooperative-Learning Strategies

What is happening to Kerry?   **Think-Pair-Share**
What is your first response?
What do you assess to correct the problem?
What medications will treat the problem?

Possible answers:
Autonomic dysreflexia; hyperreflexia
Raise the head of the bed
Assess bladder, insert Foley; assess rectum for impaction; and assess skin for burns
Apresoline and nifedipine

Reflective-Writing Prompt

Kerry's girlfriend, Anna, has visited Kerry throughout the hospitalization, but her visits have become more infrequent during rehabilitation. Kerry is becoming increasingly concerned and depressed over the situation. Write your feelings from Anna's perspective and Kerry's perspective. Does the nurse have a role in this situation?

TABLE 2.4   Case Example for Staff Development

Learning Outcomes

After processing the case, the nurse will be able to
- Describe possible solutions to dealing with an alcohol dependent peer.
- Identify ethical and legal conflicts faced when dealing with an alcohol dependent peer.

Paragraph 1

Nancy Nurse works on a surgical unit full-time evenings. She often works with Susan Nurse, who floats between evenings and nights. The last two evenings Nancy has noticed drastic changes in Susan's appearance and work habits. Susan has come to work appearing very sloppy in appearance—wrinkled uniform, runs in her hose, and mussed hair. She always seemed to be "finished" with her work and spent a lot of time in the lounge smoking. Nancy had noticed this behavior and was beginning to worry about Susan's patients.

Focused Questions and Cooperative-Learning Strategies

Group 1	What could be happening?	**Roundtable**
Group 2	What information do you need that you don't have?	**Roundtable**
Group 3	What should Nancy do?	**Roundtable** *After all three groups finish processing, they "pass the problem" to a new group and that group adds to and clarifies the list. Then, another "passes the problem." This time, the new group circles the best or most probable answers. Each group reports.

Paragraph 2

Nancy and Susan work together again. This time, Susan repeats her prior actions, but this time Nancy smells a distinctive alcoholic odor on her breath. She also notices that Susan seems shaky and unstable. Nancy asks Susan if she is OK and offers to call the supervisor for her so she could go home sick. Susan refuses, saying she cannot leave because she needs the hours and that she is just tired from "partying" last night. She promises that if Nancy does not expose her for coming to work "a little high" she'll never do it again.

Focused Questions and Cooperative-Learning Strategies

Pairs of students	What should Nancy do?	**Think-Pair-Share, then Pairs report.**
	What is the ethical dilemma?	
	What are her alternatives and possible consequences of each?	

(continued)

TABLE 2.4   Case Example for Staff Development *(Continued)*

Paragraph 3

Nancy works with Susan again, and the behavior repeats itself. She also catches Nancy "spiking" her coffee with a flask of "Southern Comfort" she conveniently keeps in her purse. Nancy confronts her and asks her to seek help through employee health. She refuses, so Nancy confides and seeks help from another staff nurse, Heather. Heather tells Nancy to mind her own business. She tells her that because she is married, she does not understand how important it is to a single person like Susan to "party" and try to find a man and a father for her 2-year-old son. She also tells Nancy to suggest to Susan to use mouthwash so no one else notices.

Focused Questions and Cooperative-Learning Strategies

Why does Heather ignore and rationalize the situation? Considering all the data, what should Nancy do?	**Roundtable and group reporting.**

Reflective-Writing Prompt

How would you feel about working with a recovered chemically dependent nurse?

---

them to fulfill their professional responsibility, protect clients, and help chemically dependent coworkers. The reflective-writing prompt stimulates the nurse to examine personal values and beliefs related to a recovered peer. Again, processing ones feelings and thoughts about an issue before experiencing it helps the nurse function more effectively when actually faced with the situation.

Unfolding Cases is a comprehensive teaching plan that allows educators to promote critical thinking, communication skills, and active involvement while promoting continuous improvement through self-reflection. Using this design, professors and staff development educators can create cases to meet specific learning outcomes, allowing students or staff nurses to be immersed in situations dealing with multifaceted data. Students come away from this experience with a sense of being able to solve complex problems with a variety of new and creative solutions. Their self-confidence is enhanced as is their ability to deal effectively with the challenges nurses face in practice. It is diverse, as is its flexibility to meet varied learning outcomes.

UNFOLDING FAMILY CASES

Unfolding Family Cases are a variation of Unfolding Cases. The elements of the case remain the same as in the unfolding case (purpose, biographical data, context, and content), but the case unfolds across the course or curriculum rather than a single class. It focuses on the individual client and the impact their problem has on their family. It provides for multiple branching of concepts or specific problems rather than a static predetermined sequence of events, which is the norm with Unfolding Cases.

In developing an Unfolding Family Case, the faculty member creates five fictional families (see Table 2.5). Students are divided into groups of five to form "primary groups." The total number of groups will depend on the number of students in the class. For example, if there are 40 students, 8 groups will be formed. Each group member is assigned a different fictional family to work with throughout the course. Periodically, "wild cards" are introduced, and students reflect in writing and discuss in groups the characteristics of the "wild card" and the impact this specific "wild card" might have on the family with which they are working.

In creating fictional families, the faculty member needs to include a variety of elements, such as culture, age, marital status, family composition, educational background, socioeconomic status, and content relevant to the objectives of the course. Table 2.5 gives an example of five such families used to teach a basic obstetrical course. It is important to create five very different families to increase the learning and broaden the scope of discussion among students.

"Wilds cards" are potential situation-specific, developmental crises or common problems that might occur in the situation created within the families. Students, in their primary groups, choose one of five cards, each depicting a different type of problem to be integrated into their fictional family. "Wild cards" are introduced periodically in the course, as new content might be in a traditional course. Figure 2.2 shows an example of how this process might proceed for one student throughout the course. This particular student selected family 1, Amy's family, to work on throughout the course. The first group of "wild cards" introduced were five potential scenarios that could occur during the first trimester of pregnancy. Note that in Figure 2.2, "normal" is used as one possible scenario as well as the problematic ones. The second set of "wild cards" presents problems of second and third trimester, and the third set of problems during labor and delivery. At selected intervals, the student would choose one of the five cards to integrate into her or his family. "Wild cards" are always drawn while students are in their "primary group" to assure a wider variance of different problems for different families. In this particular case, the student might choose "threatened abortion" first, then "pregnancy induced hypertension" (PIH), and then "premature labor." A unique sequence

TABLE 2.5   Fictional Family Examples

1   Amy Bryant is a 16-year-old Appalachian single female. She lives with her parents and six younger siblings in the "hills" of Beaver, Ohio. She attends 9th grade and has a 16-year-old boyfriend. Her family is on public assistance. She has just discovered that she is pregnant.

2   John and Irene Wong are Chinese immigrants who have recently come to the United States. They are both in their early 20s. They live in a small one-bedroom apartment above a Chinese restaurant in downtown Chicago. Both of them work at the restaurant in exchange for the apartment and a small salary. They are expecting their first child.

3   Kate McCoy and Alice Robbins are a lesbian couple who have a long-term relationship of 5 years. Kate is 38 years old and is a college Spanish professor. Alice is 42, never been married, and working as a criminal lawyer. She has hypertension and diabetes. The couple has decided to have a child together, and Kate has just found out that the artificial insemination with donor sperm has resulted in pregnancy.

4   Sarah and Jake Mullins, 44 and 48, respectively, have been married for 15 years and have had infertility problems. After trying for 10 years to become pregnant, they decided to accept the fact that they would have no children. They are financially comfortable, and both have full-time jobs, Sarah as an office manager and Jake as a marketing executive. Sarah has just found out she is pregnant.

5   Tara Cristoff is 26 years old. She has a 3-year-old son and has just gotten divorced after her husband of 4 years walked out on her. She had a one-night stand, and now she is pregnant. She is unsure if the father of the baby is the one-night stand or her ex-husband. She is getting child support but has no job at the present. She is very depressed and is afraid to tell her ex-husband that she is pregnant. Her mother lives 450 miles away and is unaware of the pregnancy or divorce.

of problems would be integrated into family 1 through this student's contributions to the group and class discussion. How the case evolves for each student will be different and depend on the cards they draw. This will create a multitude of variation, which will make for better and varied discussion in the class.

After each set of "wild cards" is drawn, students are given work to complete outside of class, on an individual basis, related to both the "problem" and the effect it may have on their family. This work is in the form of a two-part study guide asking for pertinent information on the "problem" in the first part, and a few open-ended questions to stimulate thinking as to how their particular family might react in the second part (see Table 2.6). This information is to be recorded and reflected on in writing for use in the next class.

At the next class students are grouped into "wild card groups" or groups comprising all students who have selected the same "wild

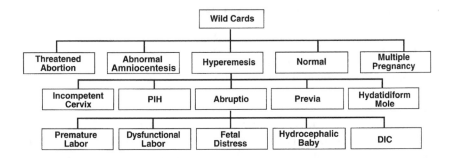

FIGURE 2.2   Amy's case unfolding.

card" but have different families. For example, all student selecting "threatened abortion" will group together. In this particular case, there will always be five different groups because there are only five different "wild cards." Yet the number of students in each group will vary, depending on the number of students in the class. If there are 40 students in the class, there will be five groups of eight each. In these "wild card" groups, they first discuss part one of the study guide and come up with a group version of answers based on the discussion and input of all students. Then the groups, using *Roundtable* (see Chapter 3), answer and discuss a set of focused questions prepared by the faculty member (see Table 2.7). A total class discussion follows as each group

TABLE 2.6   Study Guide

Part 1

1. Define the problem or condition.
2. Describe the common signs and symptoms of the problem or condition.
3. Discuss normal/abnormal laboratory data or testing needed to evaluate or diagnose.
4. Describe the usual treatment regime.
5. Describe nursing interventions appropriate in this case.
6. List possible and the most probable client outcome(s).

Part 2

1. How will your "wild card" affect your family in the following areas?
   • Feelings and reactions of family members and client (coping)
   • Communication among family members
   • Power and decision making in the family
   • Cultural implications
   • Resources and support systems
   • Potential ethical and legal dilemmas
2. What are the strengths and areas needing support in this family?

TABLE 2.7   Wild Card Group–Focused Questions

1. What are the similarities and differences in the way your family most likely reacted to this wild card problem/condition?
2. What factors contributed to the differences or similarities (culture, family composition, financial status, age, etc.)?

presents the "wild card" including answers to part 1 of the study guide and focused questions. Through class discussion, students are exposed to information on all five "wild card" problems, not just the one they drew. At this time, the faculty member can summarize important concepts, clarify and correct misconceptions, and answer questions as they arise. Important information and content are covered, but the faculty members take on the role of facilitators rather than the traditional role of experts. The student group who researched the specific topic become the ones responsible for helping other students in the class learn and comprehend the material.

The next phase of the model regroups the class into "family functioning" groups or students who selected the same family initially. These groups comprise students who have the same family but different "wild cards." Again, there will be five groups because there are five families, but the number of students in each group will vary according to the number in the class. In these groups, students using Roundtable (see Chapter 3) process another group of focused questions related to family issues dealing with the selected "wild card" problems. These are identical to the ones listed in part 2 of the study guide (see Table 2.6). Once again, a total class discussion follows as each group reports their findings to the class.

Figure 2.3 visually depicts the entire process of Unfolding Family Cases. This process can be used as the basis for an entire course, as shown in this example or as a part of a course. It has great versatility in that it can be adapted to any content area. If a family development course is being taught, the "wild cards" could be family crises or common problems families encounter as they develop. It meets requirements of the new learning paradigm in that it results in students being able to think critically, interact with others, and practice social and presentation skills. It is a vehicle that allows faculty to cover the content, yet keep students involved and interactive in the process. It also turns factual content into real-life situations and allows students to learn to solve problems of application in a safe and stimulating environment.

Again, the previous examples of Unfolding Cases and Unfolding Family Cases showed how the Comprehensive Group-Learning Model can be used in its entirety, but pieces or parts of it can be used as well.

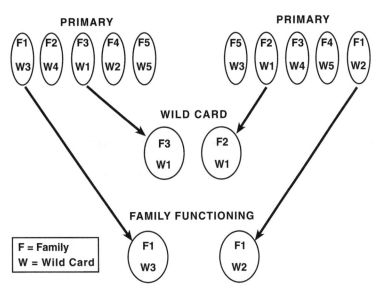

FIGURE 2.3   Student grouping for unfolding family cases.

The remainder of the book will detail specific group activities that will include selected parts of the model in various configurations. Remember, teachers select strategies that best meet their learning objectives. They can mix, match, combine, and be creative as they put these strategies to use.

CHAPTER 3

Using Cooperative-Learning Strategies in Nursing

---

ooperative-learning strategies are specific group-learning structures that help the faculty require students to be active participants in the learning process. These structures can be used
individually or combined, as the only method of teaching, or as a
break from traditional lecture methods. This chapter discusses a multitude of cooperative strategies for teachers to experiment with.

THINK-PAIR-SHARE

Think-Pair-Share is a simple classic cooperative-learning strategy developed by Frank Lyman (1987). It involves all students and is quick and
easy to implement in any class, be it a seminar of 12 or lecture hall of a
100. The professor poses a problem or question. Each student is given
60 seconds of "think" time, then students share their ideas or thoughts
about the answers to the question or problem with a peer (see Figure
3.1). At that point, each pair may report the solution to the entire class,
or selected pairs may be called on randomly to share solutions.

Using this strategy allows students time to process the task individually before sharing it with another student. Everyone must be involved,
and no one is permitted to sit passively. On sharing their individual
solutions with another student, students get both positive reinforcement
and support for their answer, which increases their confidence before

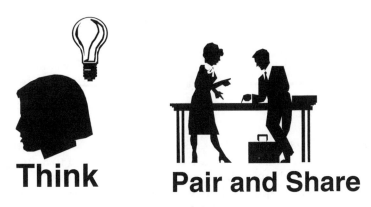

Think   **Pair and Share**

FIGURE 3.1   Cooperative strategy: Think, pair, and share.

presenting their thoughts to the whole class. Students get practice in presenting their solutions to the class, which enhances the development of their communication skills. This not only decreases their anxiety but builds their self-esteem. An additional benefit is the increased depth of learning that occurs when students must explain their ideas or solutions to another student. This requires them to analyze their own thinking processes thoroughly, an important aspect of critical thinking and reflecting. During the whole class discussion following pairs reporting to the class, professors have the chance to correct misconceptions and assess the student's depth of comprehension.

A professor might use this strategy to determine if students truly understand a complex situation or concept. For example, the professor could be lecturing on a topic such as Rh incompatibility. After the professor completes the explanation, he or she might ask students to first think about how they might explain this concept to a student who missed the class. After 1 minute of "think time," the students, in turn, explain the concept to their partner. After sharing their ideas, the professor calls on random pairs to stand and share their explanations. This gives the professor the opportunity to correct misconceptions immediately, assess the clarity of student's understanding, and reinforce the major points.

This strategy can also be used as an assessment tool periodically to ascertain student questions related to the content being presented or as a quick way to make a traditional lecture more interactive. Total time for this strategy can be as little as 5 minutes, depending on how many student pairs are called on to report. It could also be modified to include writing to give students practice in communicating. In this case, students would "think," then put their thoughts on paper or "write," and then "pair" and "share." Students could read and react to each others written thoughts, helping each understand the strengths and limitations in their ability to communicate through writing.

ROUNDTABLE

Roundtable (Kagan, 1992) is a classic cooperative-learning strategy used primarily for brainstorming. Students are assigned to a group and sit in a circular fashion while a pad of paper is passed from one student to the next. Each student verbalizes and records a possible response to the problem or question proposed by the teacher, then passes the paper to the next student. One person is then called on to report for the entire group (see Figure 3.2). It is very important that students both respond in turn and verbalize their thoughts. This prevents one or two members of the group from dominating the other members of the group and requires that everyone must participate. No one can just sit and listen. By responding verbally, each group member hears the persons' ideas and can become stimulated by those ideas, the ultimate purpose of this brainstorming exercise. One benefit of this strategy is that students soon realize the importance of preparation before coming to class as they know that they will be required to participate. Faculty members need to be sure to inform students of the content to be covered either verbally or through the syllabus, so that preparation is possible. Another benefit of working in this roundtable structure is that it encourages them to communicate with one another and helps them to begin to work in teams. Students learn important communication and social skills, such as how to include others who are often quiet in discussion, the value of hearing everyone's ideas, and the need to respect others.

Roundtable is simple to use yet produces large volumes of information. In nursing classes, instead of lecturing on signs and symptoms of a particular disease, such as increased intracranial pressure, the professor could ask students to brainstorm a list of possible signs and symptoms. Students can individually think of a couple of signs, but a long list of signs is usually formulated when students are asked to do this as a group. Once student groups report to the whole class, most signs and symptoms are reported, but if they are not faculty can add any signs or correct signs that were not appropriate. During this roundtable technique, students often feel free to ask more questions because they are stimulated by the discussion, and the technique itself invites and creates an open environment.

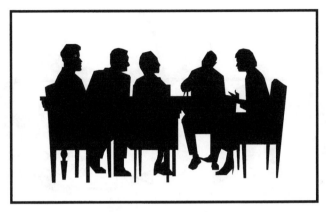

FIGURE 3.2   Cooperative strategy: Roundtable.

PASS THE PROBLEM

Pass the Problem (Kagan, 1992) usually begins with the roundtable technique in which students, in a group, process a problem or task by writing their ideas down on a sheet of paper in turn. Once their ideas are jotted down, the paper is then passed to another group of students (see Figure 3.3). When each group has a new set of ideas or solutions, they are required to clarify, prioritize, add more solutions, or whatever the teacher proposes. At this point, student groups report their solutions or they can Pass the Problem again. With the previous example, students were required to list the signs and symptoms of increased intracranial pressure. Once each group listed all of their ideas, the list is passed to another student group. The new student group could be asked to clarify the list to be sure that these are, in fact, signs of increased intracranial pressure. They could add additional signs to the list, or a teacher might ask them to identify the early and late signs of increased intracranial pressure from the list they have been passed. Reporting of these signs and symptoms, such as restlessness, vomiting, headache, pupillary changes, and Cushing's phenomena, adds to their ability to remember this factual information. When reporting their group's ideas, it also increases their understanding of priority signs and emphasizes the importance of knowing the significance of particular signs. In this example, the student might indicate that changes in level of consciousness indicate an early sign of intracranial pressure, whereas vital sign changes often indicate late signs or brainstem herniation. Through this technique students gain ideas from the previous group's brainstorming efforts and must analyze and use their powers of critical thinking to process the task.

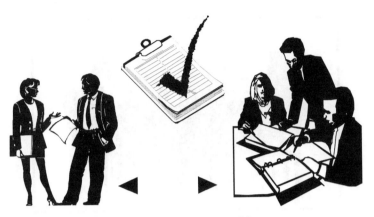

FIGURE 3.3   Cooperative strategy: Pass the problem.

JIGSAW

Jigsaw (Aronson, Blaney, Stephan, Sikes, & Snapp, 1978) is a versatile group-learning structure that presents information on a variety of related concepts. Jigsaw not only encourages students to study nursing content but also provides the opportunity for students to use the critical thinking skills of analysis, reflection, synthesis, and reconstruction (see Figure 1.3). These skills are best integrated through a cooperative-learning experience. The following example using a Jigsaw illustrates the use of these important skills (Ulrich & Glendon, 1995).

Individual students are assigned one specific nursing theory. For example, students number off from 1 to 4, and each number is assigned a different theorist. After researching and analyzing their assigned theory individually before class, students group and interact with other students who were assigned the same theory (see Figure 3.4, above the arrow). The main focus of this group's assignment is to become "experts," which requires them to answer several questions and explore a variety of concepts regarding the topic, in this case, a specific nursing theory. These questions are formulated by the professor and based on pertinent facts necessary to grasp the essence of the topic being studied. Group interaction is facilitated by using specific group learning structures. In this example, terminology used by the theorist, major concepts, application, and limitations are areas in which students must become knowledgeable to comprehend the theory.

Once students have become experts on their theory, they are regrouped so that there is one expert per theory in the new groups (see Figure 3.4, below the arrow). Each group member, in turn, explains his or her theory to the members of the new group so that all members

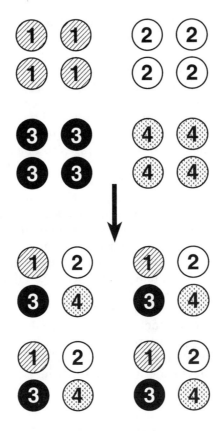

FIGURE 3.4   Cooperative strategy: Jigsaw.

become knowledgeable about each theory. Then the group creates a new theory based on knowledge gained from existing theories. The final step involves each group sharing their new theory with the entire class. See Table 3.1 for a summary of all the steps of jigsaw.

This technique promotes several critical thinking concepts. Initially, students must prepare individually, learning facts, analyzing the theory, and explaining their ideas and interpretation of the theory to others. This sharing activity encourages other group members to reflect on their own ideas and to question others' perspectives. During this process, each student's understanding of the theory is enhanced through exposure to the ideas of others. When new groups form, students gain experience in teaching others. Students must synthesize the information gained through the previous group experience and articulate this information to the new group. Finally, as the new groups develop their own theory, synthesis of all theories culminates in a reconstruction of concepts into a newly developed theory. This final step relies on knowledge of other theories but also requires students to think imaginatively.

There are numerous ways Jigsaw could be used in the nursing classroom. For example, in a management class, various ways that nursing care is delivered could be explored using this method. Groups become experts on team nursing, primary care, and case management, and ultimately design a new creative approach to care giving. As students explore the advantages and disadvantages to quality care, the cost of each method, the patient outcomes, the required patient-nurse ratio, as well as the RN and health care worker mix required, they are able to analyze methods used in nursing practice critically.

Even nursing didactic content could be taught using Jigsaw. Individuals become experts on one type of diabetes (types 1 and 2, and gestational), and then teach it to new group members using the framework of diet, exercise, and medication. Instead of Jigsaw 3, as shown in Table 3.1, students could find similarities and differences of the various kinds of diabetes, encouraging them to compare and contrast the various types. The variations are endless.

Jigsaw is a creative teaching strategy that promotes individual responsibility and group interdependence. It requires students to think critically and creatively, skills essential to practicing professional nursing. It truly meets the learning outcomes inherent in the new learning paradigm.

INSIDE-OUTSIDE CIRCLE

Inside-Outside Circle (Kagan, 1992) has many uses. It can be a structure used for team building and getting acquainted with team members or the entire class. It can be used as preparation for applying information in group class activities, reviewing for an examination, or as a means of memorizing and remembering important facts. In these situations, it is almost like a game in that students learn while moving about and having fun.

Students form two equal circles (i.e., 10 students in one circle and 10 in the other). The circles form so that one circle is inside the other one (see Figure 3.5). Students in the inside circle face outward and students in the outside circle, inward. As the circles form, each student has a partner he or she is facing. The teacher poses a factual question, such as "When do pregnant mothers experience quickening?" The pair discusses and comes to consensus on the answer. If they don't know the answer, they can ask the pair beside them. After 30 to 45 seconds

TABLE 3.1   Steps in Jigsaw

Jigsaw 1	Students study individually their assigned nursing theory before class. Students who are assigned the same theory meet and discuss pertinent knowledge relative to the theory.
Jigsaw 2	New groups are formed consisting of at least one person from each theory group. Individual members explain their theory to the other members of the group so that all members become knowledgeable about each theory.
Jigsaw 3	Using the comprehensive knowledge gained through Jigsaw 2, the group creates a new theory.
Jigsaw 4	Each group presents its theory to the entire class. Discussion follows.

From Ulrich, D., & Glendon, K. (1995). Jigsaw: A critical thinking experience. *Nurse Educator, 20*, 6–7. Reprinted with permission.

the teacher rings a bell and asks for the answer. When everyone knows the correct answer, in this case, 20 weeks, the teacher says "rotate." Inside-circle members rotate clockwise, and outside-circle members rotate counterclockwise. Each student has a new partner, and the process repeats itself.

A variation would be to give each student a 3 x 5 card, with a question on one side and the answer on the other. When they pair, they ask their partner the question on their card, praise them if they answer correctly, and show them the answer if they are incorrect or do not know. Before rotating, students exchange cards. The process repeats itself until everyone has seen all the questions.

ACADEMIC CONTROVERSY

Academic Controversy (Johnson & Johnson, 1984) is an excellent group strategy that uses intellectual conflict as the basis for learning. It is similar to a traditional debate, except that students are forced to look at both sides of an issue, not just one side. It involves analysis of the issue as well as critical thinking to find a solution to rationalize agreement with one side or the other.

The teacher selects an important intellectual issue (see Table 3.2 for examples that might be used in nursing situations). Students are put into groups of four, with two being assigned the pro position and two the con position. Then, the five-step controversy procedure described by Johnson and Johnson (1984) is followed. First, the pairs are given time to research their topic and find the best reasons for supporting

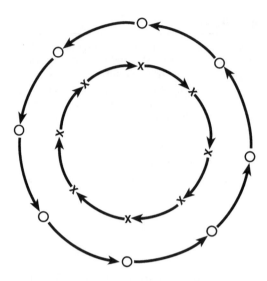

Inside circle rotates clockwise
Outside circle rotates counterclockwise

FIGURE 3.5   Inside-outside circle.

their assigned position. They also plan a way to present their position to persuade the opposing pair to their side. Second, each pair presents the case to the opposing pair. Third, in an open debate, the issue is discussed, critically evaluated, and defended by each side. Fourth, the two pairs reverse sides and present the best argument for the opposing position. Fifth, the four students drop their identified sides and discuss the issue objectively. They integrate the "best" of both sides and decide with which side they agree.

The benefits of this activity are many. Students are able to examine an issue from different perspectives and are forced to examine critically their own values and ideas for rationality. Research has consistently shown that this group activity promotes higher achievement, higher academic self-esteem, and higher quality problem-solving skills (Johnson & Johnson, 1984, 1989).

TEACHING NURSING CONTENT BY COMBINING STRATEGIES

As described by Glendon and Ulrich (1992a), the teaching plan shown in Tables 3.3 to 3.6 describes how nursing content can be taught

TABLE 3.2   Possible Nursing Topics for Academic Controversy

1. Assisted suicide is an accepted solution for consenting adults, and nurses should help if asked.
2. Fathers should have a legal right to a child before a mother chooses abortion, and if he wants the child, the mother's abortion should be denied.
3. Marijuana should be a legalized medicine as a schedule 1 drug.
4. Chemically dependent nurses should be able to practice.
5. Homosexual couples should be able to adopt children.
6. In vitro fertilization and other expensive fertility treatments should be paid for by insurance companies.
7. Organ donation should be an automatic procedure for everyone unless they have a legal document stating their objection.
8. Human cloning should be legalized.

cooperatively using multiple cooperative-learning strategies. Table 3.3 identifies the content to be covered, time allotment, and the specific student and teacher preparation before class. The student completes the assigned readings or audiovisual aid related to the topic. The teacher divides the class into heterogeneous groups of four to six members and decides on the specific cooperative strategy to be used. The professor also determines the reward for group participation and designates the grading system.

Table 3.4 describes the first cooperative strategy, Think-Pair-Share, used to identify the defining characteristics of a particular condition,

TABLE 3.3   Preparation

Content: Pregnancy-Induced Hypertension (PIH)

Student Preparation

1. Read Chapter 29, "Hypertensive States of Pregnancy," in your maternity textbook.
2. Complete the interactive videodisc on "Pregnancy-Induced Hypertension" in the computer center.

Teacher Preparation

1. Planning of assignments as stated previously.
2. Divide class into heterogeneous groups of four members and determine cooperative-learning strategies to be used.
   • Think-Pair-Share produces the defining characteristics (15 minutes).
   • Roundtable generates nursing diagnoses (15 minutes).
   • Pass The Problem brainstorms possible nursing interventions (20 minutes).
3. Teacher will quiz one member of each group and award two bonus points to each group member's next individual test grade, if answered correctly.

From Glendon, K., & Ulrich, D. (1992a). Using cooperative learning strategies. *Nurse Educator, 17,* 37–40. Reprinted with permission.

TABLE 3.4   Steps in Think-Pair-Share

- Ask students to list the defining characteristics of PIH while in their learning groups.
- Teacher allows 1 minute for each student to think individually about the defining characteristics.
- Two minutes are allowed for students to share thoughts with each other.
- Five minutes are allowed for both pairs to share thoughts with each other.
- A group list of defining characteristics evolves.
- Each group reports.
- Teacher creates a class list of defining characteristics, adding any missed items if necessary; stimulates discussion of pathophysiology and variation of disease process.

From Glendon, K., & Ulrich, D. (1992a). Using cooperative learning strategies. *Nurse Educator, 17,* 37–40. Reprinted with permission.

pregnancy-induced hypertension (PIH). This strategy allows students time to process the task and share their thoughts with another student. When the student receives positive reinforcement from a peer that high blood pressure, protein in the urine, and weight gain are the cardinal defining characteristics of PIH, confidence in participating in subsequent class discussion is enhanced. Table 3.5 explains a second cooperative strategy, Roundtable, that is used to brainstorm possible nursing diagnoses. Roundtable encourages each student to analyze a defining characteristic of PIH, such as elevated blood pressure. Then, students determine a valid nursing diagnosis for the characteristic—in this case, potential for injury related to a possible convulsion. The ability to link the defining characteristic to the appropriate nursing diagnosis is difficult for beginning nursing students, and this exercise provides the opportunity to practice this essential skill. Students soon realize the importance of preparation before class, as the strategy requires them to participate actively in turn. No one can just sit back and listen.

TABLE 3.5   Steps in Roundtable

- Using the class list of defining characteristics, each group is asked to generate a list of possible nursing diagnoses.
- Brainstorming is facilitated by requiring each student to generate a diagnosis. A pad of paper is passed in turn to each student.
- After 10 minutes, one member of each group is asked to report the diagnoses on their group list to the class.
- The teacher lists the diagnosis on the board or an overhead transparency as each group reports, suggests missed diagnoses, and promotes general discussion.

Glendon, K., & Ulrich, D. (1992a). Using cooperative learning strategies. *Nurse Educator, 17,* 37–40. Reprinted with permission.

TABLE 3.6   Steps in Pass The Problem

- Each group selects one nursing diagnosis.
- Teacher creates a folder for each selected nursing diagnosis and gives one folder to each group.
- Each group generates as many possible interventions in 10 minutes, writing interventions on paper provided in folder.
- The new group adds to and refines the existing list of interventions, creating a new list by writing on an overhead transparency provided in the folder.
- Each group reports the list of interventions related to a specific diagnosis.
- The teacher promotes discussion as the interventions are presented, suggesting interventions, and/or refining and clarifying the list.

From Glendon, K., & Ulrich, D. (1992a). Using cooperative learning strategies. *Nurse Educator, 17,* 37–40. Reprinted with permission.

However, the group that is practicing social skills tolerates error and creates an environment of acceptance, freeing the student to actively participate actively.

Table 3.6 discusses yet a third specific cooperative technique, Pass the Problem, which generates nursing interventions specific to the nursing diagnoses previously defined. Pass the Problem allows the first group of students to brainstorm a list of interventions related to a specific nursing diagnosis, such as potential for injury related to a possible convulsion. This list generally includes the obvious interventions, such as monitoring blood pressure and reflexes, administering magnesium sulfate, and instituting seizure precautions.

When passed to the second group, they add to, refine, and clarify the list. They often include additional parameters related to the blood pressure, for example, to call the physician if the blood pressure is greater than 160/100 and to position the patient on her left side. Additional interventions of measuring intake and output and assessing daily weight gains are usually identified by this second group because they must reflect on more specific details of the condition.

At the end of each strategy, the groups report their results, and the teacher verifies that the information is complete. The caliber of discussion proceeds at a higher level as students have been immersed in the material and have had time to think and reflect on the content presented.

This example, pregnancy-induced hypertension, explains how nurse educators might teach course content using multiple cooperative-learning strategies rather than traditional lecture. Essential content can be taught employing these methods, while at the same time encouraging critical thinking and practicing communication techniques in teams. Students have the opportunity to "discover" knowledge rather than "receive" it from faculty. They are active, involved, and feel connected to the material—all characteristics that promote more effective learning.

This chapter described specific cooperative–learning strategies that are used to stimulate group interaction and problem solving. Faculty members can use these strategies alone or in combination to meet their individual student-learning needs.

CHAPTER 4

Strategies to Connect Students Holistically

F aculty can stimulate students holistically through their senses, enhance critical thinking, and involve them in groups at the same time, all of which multiplies the learning potential of students. Students are tapped holistically through vision, hearing, emotions, intellect, and physical dimensions. This chapter discusses different teaching strategies and learning modalities, which can be used to stimulate memory and enhance problem-solving abilities.

DRAWINGS

Stimulating students through the use of their senses is a good way to promote learning of common signs and symptoms related to various disease states. Recognizing distinguishing characteristics of specific patient problems is a primary role of the nurse. Artwork is a unique way to bring these signs and symptoms to life and help nurses remember the many distinct clinical signs associated with a patient's disease. Drawings of a patient can slightly exaggerate the clinical characterizations in a way textbook photographs do not depict them, which helps trigger the student's memory by these visual depictions. Critical thinking related to this material can be accomplished by using specific focused questions created by the teacher to stimulate students intellectually. Questions can be formulated that encourage student analysis of the data in the artwork, or more complex questions can stimulate

41

student problem solving. This group strategy combines the use of artwork and focused questions to encourage students to apply knowledge related to a particular disease state.

Students view the picture while sitting together in a circle. After viewing the picture in detail, students, in a group, answer the questions that are found typed below the artwork. For example, Figure 4.1, a patient with Graves' disease, might be shown to the student group. After viewing the drawing, the students are asked to respond to the focused questions below the drawing. Initially, the questions should focus on the clinical manifestations shown in the drawing as well as challenge students to add additional data to the drawing by labeling common characteristics not addressed in the drawing. In this example, diarrhea, tachycardia, insomnia, and rapid speech are clinical signs not easily depicted in a drawing, whereas goiter, exophthalmos, and heat intolerance are physical signs that are apparent in the artwork. Nursing problems and their subsequent interventions require in-depth analysis of the data. Students, in their group, are then required to select three problems related to the client depicted in the artwork, and then discuss and plan nursing interventions for this client, including actual and potential problems. Once individual groups have answered all of the focused questions and designed a plan of care, a group representative shares the answers with the entire class. In this example, students might choose sleep pattern disturbance, body image disturbance, and potential for injury related to corneal injury. Students would present nursing interventions pertinent to these diagnoses. A comprehensive plan of care for the client would evolve as all groups presented their chosen nursing problems and interventions.

Artwork serves to stimulate the students' senses and encourages memory of the clinical signs. Focused questions help students use critical thinking skills to process the information by analyzing the data and determining appropriate nursing diagnoses and their interventions. Students could further be challenged by including questions that require them to establish priority or compare and contrast nursing interventions. Combining the two strategies of artwork and focused questions encourages students to remember data as well as synthesize critical questions related to specific disease states.

CONCEPT JIGSAW

Another way to use artwork and stimulate critical thinking is to combine student artwork with the cooperative-learning strategy Jigsaw (Aronson et al., 1978). The *Concept Jigsaw* is a group strategy that

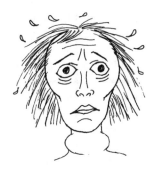

Focused Questions:

What are the clinical manifestations of Graves' disease?

What are common treatment measures?

diet _____

medications _____

Label other pertinent signs on the drawing that are descriptive of Graves' disease.

Pick 3 nursing problems and describe the nursing care.

FIGURE 4.1   Drawing of a client with Graves' disease.

helps students investigate a variety of topics within a complex concept. It is a strategy that helps the professor cover and process a variety of related topics in an organized and efficient manner. This strategy combines the basic steps of Jigsaw (see Table 3.1) and group artwork. Individual members of each student group are given different pieces of an overall concept so that within each group the total is examined in detail. Students are given study guides to direct their research into their topic and to assure that the common themes are identified and investigated. They are also asked to depict their piece of the concept visually. After individual work is completed, students come together in their group. As a group, they discuss their part, show their individual visual depictions, and become "experts" on the total topic assigned. At this point, from each individual's artwork and completed study guides, the group is asked to depict visually and label their topic in a creative way that illustrates the main features of their assigned topic. Students are stimulated intellectually to remember things better when they not only can visualize but actually physically create the depiction of important aspects of the topic. Students then regroup so that there is an "expert" on each part of each group (see Figure 3.4). In their new groups, students present their group's drawing as they explain their part, in turn, to one another. As a result, all students have been exposed to the total concept and have visualized the similarities and differences within a common group of topics. A teacher-led total class discussion completes the strategy.

For example, this strategy is an excellent way of teaching students about growth and development throughout the life span, while encouraging critical thinking about the characteristics, similarities, and differences in stages. Students are assigned to groups of five. Each group is assigned a specific developmental stage, such as infancy, toddlerhood, preschooler, school-ager, and adolescence. Within each group, individual members are assigned five different areas to research—physical characteristics, cognitive abilities, psychosocial aspects, spiritual and moral development, and health promotion and prevention needs. Individual students are given a study guide to direct them in identifying the major themes important to examine within their area. For example, the student who was assigned health promotion and prevention needs of the infant might be asked to identify the immunizations necessary for the first year of life (see Table 4.1). At the next class, students get together within their initial groups and teach their part to the rest of the group, so that this group is knowledgeable about all aspects of infancy. At this point, students, as a group, draw and label their idea of that particular developmental stage. For example, students in the infant group might draw an infant with a large head, flexed posture, fontanels, and immunizations listed with an arrow directed toward the thigh (see Figure 4.2). Students then regroup so that an "expert" on each developmental stage is in each group. "Experts" explain, discuss, and share their artwork on their assigned developmental stage. At this point, each student has been exposed to every developmental stage and is better prepared for the overall class discussion that follows. The teacher then leads an overall discussion of each developmental stage as each group shares their artwork and explains the rationale for their visual depictions. This is an excellent time to discuss variations within normal development and possible stereotypical thinking.

This strategy can also be used to discuss leadership styles, different modes of delivering nursing care, or concepts of teaching and learning. The possibilities are endless. Again, it is an excellent way to cover broad concepts quickly yet thoroughly, while actively involving students—a key to improving learning.

TABLE 4.1   Infancy—Study Guide for Concept Jigsaw

Physical	1. List characteristics about weight at 6 and 12 months. 2. When do they roll over, sit up, crawl, walk? 3. Describe eating patterns. 4. Describe elimination patterns.
Cognitive	1. Describe the outcomes of the sensorimotor period. 2. What is object permiance, and when is it likely to occur? 3. Describe the relationship between crying and infant language development.
Psychosocial	1. When do they smile? 2. What are development tasks related to Erikson? 3. What are the characteristics of bonding? 4. Describe separation anxiety, and when it is likely to occur.
Spiritual-moral	1. Give some examples of rituals specific to infancy.
Health promotion/ prevention	1. What immunizations are required during the first year? 2. What would you tell a mother about safety for this period of development? 3. What play activities/toys would you suggest for infant development?

PHOTOGRAPHS

The use of photographs and focused questions can be employed in much the same way as drawings. However, with a photograph, a real client can be used as a basis for a specific learning outcome. Similarly, focused questions can trigger problem-solving methods of students. For example, students may be shown a photograph of a client with cirrhosis of the liver. In this photograph, students could recognize the classic signs and symptoms, such as jaundice, massive ascites, everted umbilicus, dilated upper abdominal veins, and ankle edema. An initial focused question might ask, "What are the classic signs of liver disease?" Answers could include the obvious ones from the photograph or others, such as pruritus, vomiting, clay-colored stools, and coke-colored urine. A second more detailed and specific question could ask the students to cite the clinical signs specific to cirrhosis and how it differs from a patient with hepatitis A. A third question might stimulate students to explain the life-threatening complications pertaining to cirrhosis of the liver or challenge students to analyze and choose a priority nursing intervention from data given to them by faculty. With cirrhosis of the liver, students should be able to identify a potential for hemorrhage related to esophageal varices from clinical data given about the

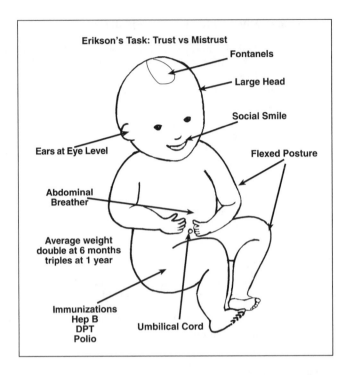

FIGURE 4.2   Example of artwork for infancy period in Concept Jigsaw.

patient's hematemesis, rapid heart rate (110), and decreased blood pressure (80/40). In a fourth variation, the teacher might also give data on two patients with liver disease, one with hepatitis A and one with cirrhosis. Students could be asked not only to compare the signs and symptoms of these liver diseases but also to analyze the differences in treatment modalities. For example, students should be able to recognize that the diet of a client with hepatitis would include protein, whereas the diet for a client with advanced cirrhosis complicated by portal system encephalopathy would require limiting the protein intake. Again, once individual groups have processed the focused questions, they share results with the entire class. At this point, a total class discussion evolves.

VIDEO, FILMS, AND TELEVISION

Video is yet another way to stimulate the senses; however, video adds the hearing and kinesthetic dimensions missing in artwork and photographs.

Students see, hear, and watch interactions, which makes the learning situation feel the most real in comparison with artwork or photographs. Video can be designed in such a way by the faculty to portray a certain message, and the information can be tailored or staged to fit the student's learning needs. If video production is too time-consuming, an alternative method of using video segments from existing commercial videotapes, feature films, or television shows can be just as effective and easy to accomplish. Focused questions are added at the designated moments in either video medium and provide the framework for student problem solving and analysis. Student groups may be challenged to view the tape and answer faculty-posed questions at either the end of the tape or at various intervals throughout the tape. Faculty can stimulate communication-related or action-oriented responses to questions. For example, "What do you think is an appropriate response or action by the nurse given the situation just viewed?" Students report their ideas, and class discussion ensues. At that point, the next segment of the video demonstrates either what the nurse said or did, or both. Students see the results of the nurse's interventions and proceed with additional processing of the current situation. Different segments can be used to process pathophysiology, pertinent nursing interventions, and communication with patients or other health team members. For example, in a faculty-produced video, a scenario of the nurse who is confronted with the client experiencing low blood sugar may be presented. The actor, as a patient, demonstrates the classic symptoms of low blood sugar—anxiety, shaking, and headache. The segment is stopped, and the instructor asks, "What could be going on with this client?" and "What should be done immediately?" At this point, groups analyze the information provided and share their analysis and solutions. The next segment of the video is shown, and the students observe that the client has indeed a low blood sugar as verified by the result of an Accucheck, and the client is given 4 ounces of orange juice. Students get immediate feedback on the appropriateness of their group's analysis and solutions. Other segments could follow with questions focusing on what could happen if treatment were not obtained or if treatment did not help, or what are other alternative interventions.

One particularly excellent videotape, *Don't Cry For Me* (Gandolfi, Tringali, & Cole, 1985) is a film highlighting the lives of adolescents with cystic fibrosis (CF). This film vividly shows the physical appearance of several different adolescents and examples of their daily regimes. Several adolescents discuss their thoughts and feelings about having CF. The teacher stops the video at various intervals and asks groups to answer pertinent focused questions regarding the segment. The learning is compounded by tapping students holistically through viewing and hearing the segments and the critical thinking required of the focused questions. Two other excellent films are *Living With AIDS* (DiFelician-tonio, 1986), a film about a young, white homosexual man; and *Special Care* (Centre Productions, 1984), a film about children born prematurely and their diverse experiences in the neonatal intensive care unit. Faculty could also use television series or feature films to help students evaluate family-processing or cultural differences. Students, in groups, view several episodes of a particular show or an entire feature film and complete a family assessment and care plan based on family theory. For example, students might view *Roseanne, Grace Under Fire,* or the film *Parenthood* as the basis for the process (Ulrich, Teets, & Quinn, 1994). Students could also analyze a *Star Trek* episode depicting communication patterns, cultural norms, and interactional patterns associated with characters from the different planets. After viewing the episode, students, in groups, could be asked to respond to focused questions, such as "Were the communities of these two different cultures competitive or cooperative?" and "How were the communication patterns of the two cultures similar or different?" In this way, students can vividly recognize these differences that will help them recognize subtler differences in existing cultures.

SIMULATION

Simulation is another way to stimulate the senses and evoke critical thinking. Student pairs could be asked to view a typical simulated hospital room. The room would have a client sleeping in a hospital bed. The room would be set up to mock several safety hazards. These hazards might include such things as the Foley bag touching the floor, uncapped syringes lying at the bedside, the bed in high position, and side rails down. When asked, "What's wrong with this scene?" each student pair will generate a list of the problems they identify. The total class then reconvenes, and each pair shares the findings as the instructor records the hazards on the board. As each hazard is identified, the instructor discusses the significance of the hazard and encourages student pairs to think of ways to prevent the hazard from occurring. Other ways to extend the learning are for faculty to propose focused questions that challenge students to think of ways to manage these breaks in safety standards.

Variations of this strategy might include having the students imagine the client in a different developmental stage, such as a child or an elderly client. Critical thinking is enhanced further by adding information and changing the focused questions to things, such as "What is missing in the mock scene?" or "What is the first thing the nurse should do when he or she enters the room?" Faculty could also add additional information about the client, such as labatory results, or recent nurses' notes to make the situation more complex and extend the critical thinking process. For example, a sample scenario of a child with a tonsillectomy could challenge the students to study the environment and identify the need for the Yanker suction equipment at the bedside. Simulations create a sense of reality yet allows faculty to encourage problem solving without the risk of client injury.

Simulation is a good way to ensure student's comprehension of the principles involved in dressing changes, catheter insertion, intravenous administration, medication administration, and other skill-related tasks involved in the nursing role. Faculty can demonstrate the skill involved incorrectly in front of a group of students. The group is challenged to critique and list all the breaks in technique on the board or overhead. After the demonstration, the group members are asked to list all of the principles that must be followed while performing the skill they just observed. Then, using the list of errors, identify which principles were violated by the faculty member. Two benefits of this technique are that the faculty member makes the errors instead of the student, which puts students more at ease in their novice state. Also, it encourages them to use critical thinking about the principles involved in the skill rather than memorizing a step-by-step approach to learning the nursing task.

EMPATHY EXPERIENCES

Empathy experiences connect students' feelings and emotions related to the patient and the situation and stimulates a deeper learning. Faculty tap the students' emotions in these experiences and stimulate them to imagine the perspective of another person.

Nurses are called to care for individuals with problems and life experiences that are often vastly different from their own. Planning experiences that build insight into the patient's unique needs helps the student to move from feeling only sympathy for the patient to having empathy or understanding. Ultimately, this understanding leads the nurse to help the patient set realistic goals. Activities that put the student nurse into the position of feeling what it is like to be ill, homeless, disabled, or different from others kindles the development of insight into the patient's needs and begins to instill a foundation for caring, which is essential to nursing practice.

There are several commonly used ways to place students in this unique position and help them get a glimpse of what it might feel like to be a patient. Student groups are assigned to explore an empathy experience. Students choose to pretend to be a diabetic for a day by following a prescribed diet and sticking themselves for blood sugars, spend a day in a wheelchair, or wear socks over their hands to simulate a physical disability. It also may require them to perform activities like eating, writing, or buttoning their clothes while simulating the disability. Placing students in pairs works best for this experience. One student experiences the activity, and the other student observes or takes on the role of frustrating the other student with obstacles or negative comments, such as, "hurry up, we're late." In contrast, the observer could also take the role of helping the student patient feel accepted. Students should be cautioned that this is a pretend activity, and safety precautions must be taken as indicated by the activity. Students could be given the choice of this activity or another assignment. In other words, the student volunteers to participate, as developing caring requires a desire by the student to truly experience this feeling state. Other activities that could be substituted are interviewing or spending the day with someone who is disabled, chronically ill, or wheelchair bound.

Once each student pair has completed the experience, the pair returns to the group. The entire group shares their experiences with each other and decides on a way to present ideas, experiences, and insights to the whole class. For example, this could be accomplished with a paper, poster, presentation, poem, quilt, or other artistic expressions. In this way, students are exposed to a variety of feeling states through the eyes of others.

FISH BONE

The *Fish Bone* strategy (Ishikawa, 1982) is a cognitive problem-solving structure that has frequently been used in the business field and is easily adapted to the educational setting. It is a useful technique that educators can use to stimulate critical thinking among students and at the same time promote the concepts of teamwork and cooperation, skills essential in professional nursing. Learning this strategy is especially beneficial because, as practicing nurses, students will be expected to use this problem-solving method when they are members of continuous quality improvement teams, a concept popular and pervasive in the work world.

To apply the Fish Bone strategy, faculty members assign students to heterogeneous groups of four to five members. The professor poses a problem and the groups must identify the potential cause of this problem, using the Fish Bone diagram (see Figure 4.3), which illustrates a cause-and-effect relationship. The groups brainstorm a list of potential causes for the problem. Ishikawa (1982), the original creator of Fish Bone, used four general areas under which to categorize the causes: people, methods, material/supplies, and equipment to stimulate the group's brainstorming. Categories are meant to prompt student thinking, not limit the brainstorming process. If desired, the professor can eliminate the categories to encourage the free flow of ideas. There are several ways to record the group's ideas. As ideas are generated, the blackboard in the classroom could be used, or students could use a pad of paper on which to draw the Fish Bone and record the information in turn. Another especially useful tool is the use of "Post-It Notes" to record ideas. These are good to use because they can easily be moved around on the diagram, which is important when combining the like causes, the next step in the process. Students often contribute the same idea, although perhaps in different words, so identical causes can be combined, and the group can come up with one "Post-It," incorporating all similar ideas for the Fish Bone. Brainstorming should not be stopped to settle these issues, but collated in the second step of the process, after brainstorming is complete.

As described by Ulrich and Glendon (1994), the professor could pose the problem that "the number of people contracting the AIDS virus continues to increase, despite an increased awareness of the disease." In completing the diagram, under the category of "people" (if categories are being used), students might list "unsafe sex practices continue to exist" as a cause of the problem. If individual students report a similar idea, then these are clarified and combined in the second step by asking these students if their idea has a uniquely different meaning. After causes are determined, students must be encouraged to include subcauses on the diagram. Subcauses often lead to uncovering the actual root cause of a problem. A way to elicit these subcauses is to encourage students to ask the "why" question of the cause generated: "Why do unsafe sex practices continue to exist?" In this case, two subcauses might include "the attitude that people believe they will not contract AIDS or a lack of accurate knowledge regarding the spread of the disease exists." Students should be encouraged to continue to ask the "why" question of these subcauses until answers are exhausted. Similarly, subcauses should be investigated with all other causes that were previously generated. Finally, through group consensus, the group circles the potential root cause for further investigation. In this example, students, by consensus, might circle the root cause, "the attitude that people believe they will not contract AIDS." Students would

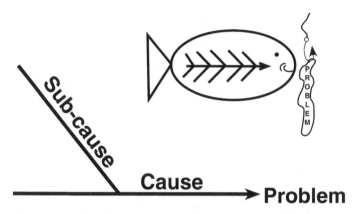

FIGURE 4.3   Fish Bone diagram. From Ulrich, D., & Glendon, K. (1994). Fishbone strategy: A TQM strategy applied to nursing education. *Nurse Educator, 19,* 7–8. Reprinted with permission.

then be encouraged to do further study using objective methods to validate that this is actually the root cause of the problem. To complete this strategy, students would need to collect data to verify the root cause circled. In this case, students might conduct a survey of student attitudes about contracting AIDS. Once the root cause is identified, students could determine appropriate solutions to this societal problem based on facts, not intuition. Instructors can adapt this tool to students' educational needs by interrupting this process at any point to engage students in class discussion or debate. Figure 4.4 summarizes the steps of the Fish Bone strategy.

The Fish Bone is a versatile strategy that can be adapted to many nursing situations with students or staff. Staff nurses could brainstorm a list of problems using the Roundtable technique on their unit, reserving some for study with the Fish Bone strategy. As described by Glendon and Ulrich (1992b), each member of each group volunteers and writes down a problem they have experienced on a pad of paper as it is passed from one to another in turn. This ensures that each staff member contributes, and active participation becomes the norm. Common problems that usually surface during this exercise include inequitable assignments, short staffing, quality assurance problems, cost-containment issues, incomplete shift reports, and patient care dilemmas, to name a few. During this process groups learn and practice social relationship skills that create an environment of acceptance and respect for every member's contribution, which, in turn, increases individual self-esteem and acceptance. Each group then selects one of

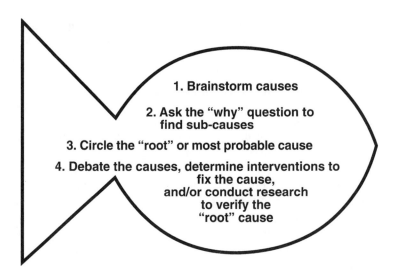

FIGURE 4.4   Steps of Fish Bone strategy.

these identified problems to analyze using Fish Bone. Through the use of a visual fishbone diagram, the groups brainstorm to list potential causes in relation to four general categories on the diagram (people, methods/protocols, materials/supplies, or equipment). These categories help trigger critical thinking related to possible causes. All categories may not be complete, as not every category is germane to every problem. After completing their brainstorming and grouping of like causes, groups, through consensus, circle the most likely root cause for further investigation. For example, a group might choose "inequitable assignments" as a problem. Under the category of "people," staff members might list unequal skill levels of staff as a possible causative factor. Under the category of "methods or unit protocols," group members could list that the charge nurses are the only assignment makers. Inclusion of any potential subcauses that might exist is critical to the process. One subcause of the example, the charge nurse on each shift is the only assignment maker, could be that the charge nurses lack skills in assignment making, or skill levels are inconsistent among charge nurses. A thorough analysis helps the staff to decide the likely root cause on their unit. If the charge nurse is viewed as the main cause of the problem, it is circled on the diagram, and the group's task is complete for this strategy. An additional step of collecting quantitative data is needed to validate this root cause before continuing to the intervention phase. For example, surveying of nurses on all shifts could be done to validate this particular example.

Next, using Pass the Problem (Kagan, 1992), nurses generate interventions to solve the problem based on the identified root cause. The manager collects each group's fish bone and places each one in a separate folder. The folders are then distributed randomly to groups who decide on possible interventions related to the root cause of each problem. The folders, complete with interventions, are then passed to another group that adds to and refines the existing list. For example, with the problem of "inequitable assignments," the list of interventions related to the root cause (charge nurse as sole assignment maker) might include rotating choice of assignments, rotating assignment maker, dividing assignment to achieve a balanced patient acuity, choice of keeping assignment for consecutive days, training of charge nurses, or collaborative assignment making. The manager promotes discussion as the interventions are presented and allows staff to reach agreement on interventions to implement. Once the intervention is decided, the manager and staff agree on a period for trial use of the intervention and schedule another team session to evaluate the intervention. When cooperative strategies are used, individual nurses become aware of their importance to the unit. They develop a sense of interdependence and increase their level of personal responsibility to the unit (Aumiller & Rudloff, 1986). This meaningful involvement is an internal motivator that transforms the nurse from a mere worker to a committed, satisfied, and involved member of the organization (see Figure 4.5). Workers who feel ownership, coupled with increased autonomy and responsibility, feel compelled to improve the quality of their performance—in this case, the overall quality of patient care.

As nurses, it is becoming vital that we learn to analyze problems readily and develop innovative interventions based on factual data. The Fish Bone strategy helps students identify root causes that lead to pinpointing more effective solutions to problems. It connects students cognitively and requires them to think critically and use creative problem-solving techniques.

CONCEPT MAPPING

Dewey (1944), early on, recognized that learning involved making linkages between what the student already knows and new information. Concept maps take this idea of creating linkages and use it as a cognitive structure to help students advance their learning. Before the development of their own concept map, students may be shown an example of a simple concept map to familiarize and help them gain confidence in their ability to create their own maps (Beitz, 1997).

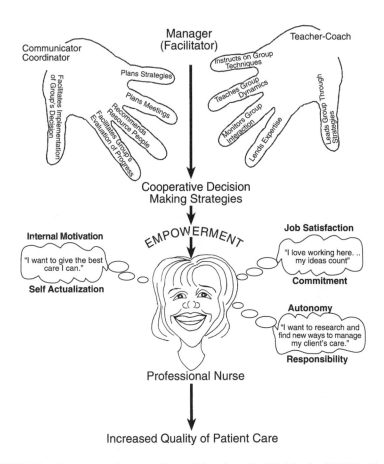

Cooperative Decision
Making Strategies

Increased Quality of Patient Care

FIGURE 4.5   Empowered nurse. From Glendon, K., Ulrich, D. (1992b). Using cooperative decision making strategies in nursing practice. *Nursing Administration Quarterly, 17,* 69–73. Reprinted with permission.

Figure 4.6 is an example of a simple concept map that could be shared with students. It is important to emphasize that there are no wrong ways to conceptualize concepts and that concept maps may look very different, depending on the depth of understanding the student possesses. Clinical practice is an excellent area in which to demonstrate use of this cognitive structure (Daley, 1996). A good place to begin is on the first day of clinical. The concept map helps students visually diagram the process of clinical preparation and what it entails. Faculty can distribute a handout that lists on the top of the page the name of the patient, age, and diagnosis followed by an arrow pointing downward. (These assignments could be actual or fictional.) The next statement is

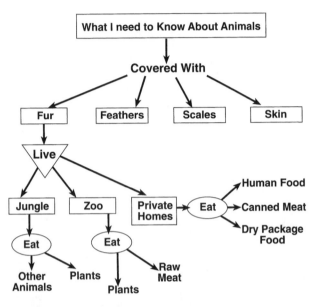

FIGURE 4.6   Simple concept map.

a prompt to help the student begin this process and says, "what I need to know." The students' first work is to diagram individually what they need to know related to their own assignment and then to consult with their group members to process jointly each student's individual patient assignment. Figure 4.7 shows an example of one student's concept map.

By diagramming linkages between what they know and think about what they should know, students gain insight into the whole experience. Early concept maps should show that students lack ability to recognize everything they need to know before beginning patient care. As in Figure 4.7, this student got a lot of information from the chart but missed data from patient interview, previous nurse, and family members. As Daley's (1996) research concluded, students often fail to link knowledge from books or classroom related to medications, patient diagnosis, and abnormal assessment data. By having students first develop their own concept maps, and then as groups discuss and build on individual maps, students are better prepared for clinical than if no group discussion occurred. Perhaps when these students share their maps with other group members, they will realize on their own where their deficits lie and be able, as a group, to come up with a more complete and accurate guide for preparing for patient care.

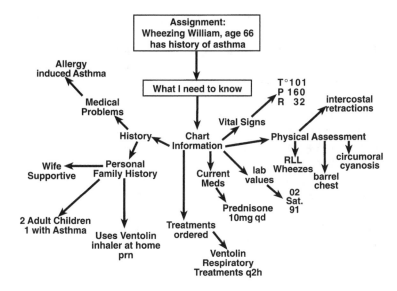

FIGURE 4.7   Patient assignment concept map.

Students need to be taught how to prepare—it is not a skill that is instinctual. Concept maps help them to integrate all of the things they need to know in an organized manner. It allows them to visualize their own thinking processes and helps them analyze how they have developed their plan in preparing for patient care.

FLOW CHARTING

A similar concept, yet different from concept mapping, is flow charting. Flow charting requires the student to look at an entire process by breaking it down into small sequential steps. As they examine each step, students are forced to question the need and value of it, thereby stimulating their intellectual processes. On completion of the flow chart, students not only understand the process more completely but have synthesized the knowledge of one process and are better able to apply it to another situation. A flow chart is a visual depiction of a procedure. It traces individual steps, provides a standard, and ensures a consistent plan for implementation. This visual conceptualization provides a reference for people who are unsure of the process, promotes quality by encouraging analysis that stimulates the continuous improvement process, and saves time by eliminating costly trial-and-error methods common in processes that are not well established.

Students in groups could be assigned a procedure to flow chart. In the clinical area, it may be a procedure that students have previously done, have observed staff nurses doing, or something that they will be required to do that particular clinical day. By completing the flow chart, students will better understand the process as well as the rationale for each step. It will serve as a better preparation method than merely reading the steps from a procedure book. Visualization of the process will stimulate their memory of key parts of the overall process. Figure 4.8 shows a completed flow chart depicting the process of drawing up a medication for intramuscular injection. By completing this process as a group, all students become familiar with all the elements of preparing a medication for injection. They may find time-saving and safety-related strategies to improve this procedure that are not apparent to nurses completing this task on a routine basis. Students are required to think and use their intellectual and cognitive abilities to connect with the learning.

CONCEPT CASE ANALYSIS

Concept case analysis is a cognitive structure in which students are given a case situation and asked to pull from the case data, illustrating a specific concept. Students are also asked to develop interventions related to the data. Student groups are given a case as well as a chart outlining specific information to be retrieved from the case. Students must fill in the data, first finding specifics in the case illustrating various parts of the concept, then determining appropriate interventions relevant to the client needs. Tables 4.2 and 4.3 shows an example using

TABLE 4.2   Concept Case Analysis

Case

Alice Williams is a 32-year-old white woman diagnosed with rheumatoid arthritis. She is 5 feet, 8 inches tall and weighs 110 pounds. She is a single mother with two preschoolers. She has been on bedrest for 3 weeks complaining of severe pain with any movement of her right ankle, left patella, and severe redness and swelling in the sacral area. Recently, she has been complaining of abdominal pain. Today's vital signs are T101, P120, R32, and BP 90/50.

Doctor's Orders

Naproxen, 375 mg tid
Plaquenil, 200 mg qd
Prednisone, 10 mg bid
Bactrim DS i hs
Iron Dextran 100 mg IM
Chair tid for 30 minutes

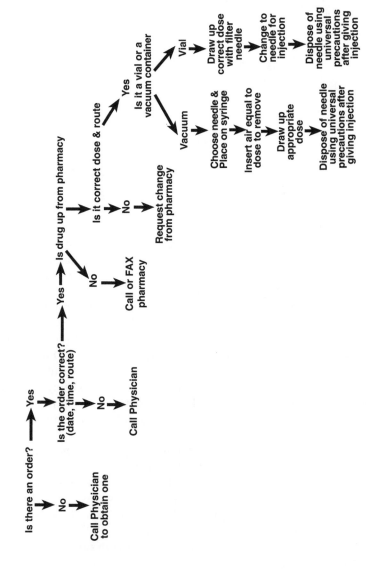

FIGURE 4.8 Flowchart for IM injection.

Is there an order? → Yes

No ↓
Call Physician to obtain one

Is the order correct? (date, time, route) → Yes → Is drug up from pharmacy

No ↓
Call Physician

Is drug up from pharmacy → Yes → Is it correct dose & route

No ↓
Call or FAX pharmacy

Is it correct dose & route → Yes → Is it a vial or a vacuum container

No ↓
Request change from pharmacy

Is it a vial or a vacuum container → Vial → Draw up correct dose with filter needle → Change to needle for injection → Dispose of needle using universal precautions after giving injection

Is it a vial or a vacuum container → Vacuum → Choose needle & Place on syringe → Insert air equal to dose to remove → Draw up appropriate dose → Dispose of needle using universal precautions after giving injection

59

TABLE 4.3   Concept Case Analysis Chart

	Hazards of Immobility	
System/hazards	Data in the case	Nursing interventions
Musculoskeletal		
Integumentary		
Cardiovascular		
Respiratory		
Genitourinary		
Gastrointestinal		
Psychological		
Nutrition		

the concept of hazards of immobility in the case of a 32-year-old woman with rheumatoid arthritis. Students would first be challenged by the professor to discuss and complete the column "System/hazards" by listing common findings in this category. For example, under "Cardiovascular," common findings related to immobility are increased heart rate and orthostatic hypotension. Next, faculty should ask students to find data in the case related to the hazards of immobility related to the cardiovascular system. Students would identify increased heart rate (120) and a low blood pressure (90/50) as significant findings for this category. In completing the intervention column, students should identify the potential risk of orthostatic hypotension and institute nursing measures of taking blood pressure in a lying and then sitting position, and then having the patient dangle her legs before getting out of bed. Students will be stimulated to find all the data and nursing implications related to this example.

Virtually any concept could be taken in its parts and used similarly in a case situation. For example, aspects of caring, components of self-concept, types of stress, functional patterns, or safety hazards are a few concepts that work well with cases. This strategy helps students structure their thinking and analytic skills as well as allows them to work together to enhance the depth of learning.

This chapter described ways faculty can make deeper connections with students by stimulating them through their senses. Students are connected holistically by intellectual, emotional, physical, visual, and auditory dimensions. These activities serve to allow them to experience the world through various mediums.

CHAPTER 5

Group Structures for Preparation and Review

If we expect students to think critically and reflect on their own learning, we must first assure that they have the factual information they need to achieve these higher level thinking skills. Preparation becomes a major part of the learning equation. How can we as faculty assure they are prepared to participate in the group-learning strategies we design? We need to give meaningful preparatory homework assignments that give them at least a first exposure to the material we deem as vital for their learning. This chapter details numerous activities and games that not only help students learn and remember information but also help them review for tests, licensure examinations, and certification requirements.

STUDY GUIDES

One way faculty can help students discriminate when they read or view videos is to require the completion of a study guide before the class. Study guides are effective ways for students to think about the material individually and try to understand and put the content into a meaningful context for themselves. The study guide contains questions written by faculty that encourage students to reflect on the important aspects of the content and focus the student's attention to this vital material (see Table 5.1). Study guides written by textbook authors are also useful, but faculty members may want to modify both the length and content in these guides to meet their own learning objectives.

Another benefit of the study guide is that it makes the student individually accountable for learning pertinent facts before class. Students

TABLE 5.1   Example of a Study Guide for Cystic Fibrosis

Cystic Fibrosis (CF) (Whaley & Wong, 1993, pp. 742–747)

1. What is the incidence of CF?
2. What culture is primarily affected?
3. Because this is a genetic, autosomal recessive disease, what is the chance of two people with the trait conceiving a child with CF?
4. What is the estimated life expectancy of children with CF?
5. What is the basic clinical feature of CF?
6. Describe how the functional patterns are affected by CF.

Activity Exercise

What respiratory assessments are common?
What treatments can the nurse perform to loosen secretions?
What common drugs are administered to reduce infectious processes?
Describe the teaching parents will need related to central lines, venous access ports for home care.
What other respiratory treatments will parents need to learn to manage?
How does hot weather and exercise influence children with CF?

Nutrition-Metabolic

Why do these children have poor weight gain and a thin, underdeveloped appearance?
What medications are used to enhance nutritional absorption?
What supplemental feedings are generally used at night?
Describe the teaching needed for parents/child related to nasogastric or nasojejunal tube feedings.
What contributes to the bleeding tendency in the child with advanced CF disease?
What disease leads to additional nutrition problems in a child with advanced disease?

Role Relationship

How can nurses support families experiencing CF?

Self-Perception

Explain how individuals are affected by this disease.
What is the effect of having CF on development, especially adolescence?
What interventions can nurses encourage to influence a positive self-concept?

Elimination

What assessment is critical in newborns to monitor for this problem early on?
What are the characteristics of stools?
Why is there an increased chance of bowel obstruction and prolapse of the rectum?

realize early on that the teacher's role is one of helping students process, apply, and make meaning of facts and information, not repeat information available in a book or on a videotape. Faculty can stimulate accountability by giving points for completion of this activity or requiring these guides for admittance into class. Study guides also assure that the students' first exposure to the material occurs before class. This allows students to process the material in class through cases or other problem-based strategies, where students are able to apply facts, question, and discuss issues at a more in-depth level. They also can get help in class as they try to use the information, a time when many students need the faculty's expertise. Essentially, this preparation results in a higher level of learning.

Even if faculty members have reduced the amounts of information they expect students to know and helped students to discriminate essential from "nice-to-know" concepts, it is important to remember that information is still difficult for some. Games are an effective way to help students remember facts by actively involving them in activities that make learning fun and interactive.

GAMES THAT STIMULATE MEMORY AND ENHANCE LEARNING

Gaming structures meet all the necessary elements for learning nursing content. Television game shows, board games, and crossword puzzles can provide the basic steps in conducting the game and can be adapted to reinforce recall of essential information before in-depth discussion in class. This eliminates the need for educators to review facts in a lecture, and reserves the time in class for processing of nursing content in relation to clinical situations.

Games are also adaptable for use in different educational settings. Staff nurses who need yearly reviews regarding policies, standards, or basic competencies of the institution could be taught to review this content through gaming. Staff might be challenged with procedural information related to special medications commonly used in intensive care or points pertinent to remember about the policy of the institution on fire safety.

Student nurses enjoy games before testing of content or for National Council Licensure Examination (NCLEX) review. These games help students prepare, process, recall, and remember information before tests by actively involving them in groups. Games stimulate students' thinking about the material and in so doing lead them to ask questions to satisfy their own learning needs.

TIC-TAC TEST READY (Glendon & Ulrich, 1995)

As described by Glendon and Ulrich (1995), this game can be used with a small seminar of 15 students, or it can be adapted to larger classes. Each student's assignment before class is to review all reading and class notes on which they are to be tested and develop at least one test question per reading assignment or class period. Question format can vary as long as the response can be given verbally in a few words (true/false, fill in the blank, simple listing, multiple choice, etc.). The questions should reflect the most important content and be written on separate index cards and brought to class the day of the game. On game day, students are divided into five groups of three students each, providing there are only 15 students in the class. Before starting the game, each of the groups is required to take a portion of the questions, analyze them, delete any inappropriately stated questions, or modify them to read correctly. This is an important step in the process because students frequently lack skill in constructing test questions and by reviewing them as a group the questions become more succinct and pertinent. This activity also helps students analyze test questions and understand the reasoning behind the answer. Next, three of the five groups combine to form the nine squares of the tic-tac-toe board, which is drawn on the blackboard or overhead. Each of the nine students places his or her name in one of the squares. The remaining two groups (six students) compete in playing the traditional tic-tac-toe game. The professor serves as the game show host, score keeper, and judge. If the class is larger, students could be assigned these roles rather than the professor. Also, pairs of students rather than individual students could form the nine squares of the tic-tac-toe board, and the two groups playing the game could be larger than three students.

The game begins with a coin toss to determine which team goes first. The first team selects a square, and the person designated in that square asks the team one of their questions. The team has 1 minute to confer on the answer and respond. The student who researched the question validates the correctness of the answer. If this student misunderstands the material, the professor overrules the decision and explains the rationale for the correct answer. If the question is answered correctly, the team places an X in that square. If the team is incorrect, the opposing team is required to answer the same question correctly to place an O in the square. If neither team answers the question correctly, the square remains blank, and the judge explains the correct answer to the missed question. Teams take turns choosing squares, and the game continues until one team wins either three Xs or three Os in a straight or diagonal line. Rotation of team players and squares occurs at varying intervals, every two or three games, and continues until all the questions are exhausted or the class period ends.

As previously stated, this game can be played with many students by using teams to serve as the judge and teams to form the squares rather than individuals. Increasing the number of students on the teams who are the players also is a way to adapt the game to a larger group of students.

Because this is a game, prizes add to the competitive spirit and fun of the activity. The authors use candy to reward the winners; however, rewards also could include buttons; nursing professional supplies, such as pen lights and scissors; or even bonus points on tests. However, the use of bonus points is a controversial issue, and individual teachers need to determine the rewards appropriate for the activity.

LET'S PLAY NURSE (Ulrich & Glendon, 1997)

This game is based on the ideas and rules of "Bingo" and is used as a method for test review, although it could also be used as an overall NCLEX review. Students learn pertinent content and prepare for testing, yet enjoy themselves in the process.

As described by Ulrich and Glendon (1997), the first step in creating the game is to plan and write a variety of questions based on the same criteria used in planning any test. A good plan might be to model the test blueprint after the NCLEX format with questions on steps of the nursing process as well as questions related to safety, physiological integrity, psychosocial integrity, and health promotion. All questions need to have relatively short answers, yet incorporate analysis and application as well as recall (see Table 5.2). At least 100 questions written on 3- x 5-inch cards with the question on one side and the answer on the other are needed for a typical game. Faculty develop the questions for this game; however, students could create the questions as they study the content, which would compound the learning potential of the game. All of the question cards are placed in a large fishbowl in preparation for the student game.

The next step requires creating the nurse cards, much like Bingo cards (see Table 5.3). In creating the nurse cards, faculty randomly select question cards from the bowl and sequentially write one answer in each of the empty boxes on the nurse card. After returning the questions to the fishbowl, the same procedure is repeated to create each new nurse card. As many cards as needed for teams to play are developed. For example, in a class of 30 students, there could be six teams of five players each; therefore, the teacher would need six different nurse cards for the game.

Students are then divided into teams. Each team is given a nurse card. Questions are drawn from the fishbowl by the instructor or another student and posed to all teams. Teams are given 1 minute to

TABLE 5.2   Questions for "Let's Play Nurse" Game

I. *Analysis/Application*

1. A woman with placenta previa is admitted to Labor & Delivery. Assessment data show fetal heart rate of 100 and maternal BP of 80/40. What do you anticipate is happening?
Answer: hemorrhage

2. Maria is 36-weeks pregnant, states her baby is not moving, and is scheduled for an non-stress test (NST). If the NST is nonreactive, what would you anticipate will happen next?
Answer: contraction stress test (CST)

II. *Recall*

1. Symptoms of pregnancy induced hypertension (PIH) include elevated blood pressure, edema, and_____.
Answer: proteinuria

2. Symptoms are painless, bright red vaginal bleeding in the third trimester that increases in amount with each episode of bleeding.
Answer: placenta previa

From Ulrich, D., & Glendon, K. (1997). Let's play nurse. *Nurse Educator, 22*(6), 9–10. Reprinted with permission.

discuss possible answers with their teammates. At that point, one team is called on to present their answers to the question, generating a full class discussion. Only teams with the correct answer on their card are permitted to mark them. This process continues until one team yells "nurse," indicating a win with five correct answers in a row either on the diagonal, horizontal, vertical, or all four corners (see Table 5.4). In a final examination review, a coverall card could be required for a nurse win.

CROSSWORD PUZZLE COMPETITIONS

Crossword puzzles can be designed to cover information related to pathophysiology, knowledge of medications, or even nursing theorists. A strategy to make factual learning interesting and fun is to make completion of the puzzle a competition between student groups. For example, instead of the teacher lecturing on the three Ps of diabetes—polyuria, polydipsia, and polyphagia—a crossword containing this information is used at the beginning of the class. Several minutes, as determined by the length of the puzzle, are allowed for student groups to finish their puzzle. It is optimal to either pair or use groups of three for this activity, as students need to be able to readily see the puzzle's across and down statements while sitting together and having only one puzzle. Once a student group is finished with the puzzle, those in the

TABLE 5.3   Sample Nurse Card

N	U	R	S	E
		FREE		

group raise their hands, or to add to the lively spirit of the game, groups could design their own signal to indicate completion of the task. To quickly verify correctness of the answer, the teacher uses an overhead transparency of a completed crossword and overlays the transparency on the student's answer sheet. If incorrect answers are detected, the game continues until another group accurately completes the puzzle. The first team that completes the puzzle correctly earns a prize as determined by the faculty.

Puzzle design is easily accomplished by creating statements for both the "across" and "down" sections of the puzzle and their answers. Computer programs are now available that automatically create the word blocks of the crossword, so most of the work lies in thinking about how to formulate the statements to fit a particular one-word answer. Examples of crosswords related to multiple topics are found in the current literature (Galuska, 1995; Lenaghan, 1996), or faculty members could devise their own (see Tables 5.5 and 5.6).

CROSSWORD COLLABORATIONS AND GRAND FINALE

Another variation on this same theme of using crosswords is to allow students to collaborate on the puzzles but eliminate the competitiveness of the game. Students collaborate in pairs or groups of three at the beginning of class on a crossword pertaining to previous reading

TABLE 5.4   Sample of a Vertical Win Nurse Card

N	U	R	S	E
Muscle tone	Rhogam	Pregnancy Induced Hypertension (PIH)	Contraction Stress Test (CST)	Respirations
Elevated temperature	Abruptio placenta	Vaginal examinations	Pale or blue color	Apnea and bradycardia
Tachycardia	Neural tube defect	Free	Trendelenburg	Painless vaginal bleeding
Lecithin/ Sphingomyelin Ratio (L/S ratio)	Gavage	Painful vaginal bleeding	Broncho-pulmonary dysplasia (BPD)	Amniocentesis
Non Stress Test (NST)	Placenta previa	Give calcium gluconate	Right occiput posterior (ROP)	Fetal lung maturity

From Ulrich, D., & Glendon, K. (1997). Let's play nurse. *Nurse Educator, 22*(6), 9–10. Adapted with permission.

assignments and the class content for the day. After a specified amount of time, faculty displays answers on an overhead transparency for students to check their results and make any corrections. Each week, a crossword is used to begin the class. By the end of the course, students have collected multiple crosswords containing essential facts that are of great use for test review. By using crosswords, faculty encourages the student to be involved in learning important facts and processing this necessary information prior to class discussion. This activity enhances the student's memory of the content and stimulates them to ask questions when class time begins. At the completion of the course, a portion of the final examination includes a comprehensive crossword puzzle including a sample from each of the previously used crosswords. The use of this strategy helps students memorize important definitions and concepts that are needed before being required to apply the information to clinical nursing situations.

ULTIMATE MEMORY GAME

This game is based on the memory game of "Concentration." In the traditional game, the player turns over a playing piece and matches it to

TABLE 5.5   Crossword Puzzle for Neurological Assessment

1	2	3	4	5	6	7	8	9	10	11	12	13	14	15	16
										R					
								V	A	L	S	A	L	V	A
D	E	C	A	D	R	O	N			C	P				
						A				C	I				
B	R	U	D	Z	I	N	S	K	I	O	N				
						O				O	A				
						A	S	P	I	R	I	N	L	F	
						H								A	
						A							C		C
			C	A	R	B	O	N	D	I	O	X	I	D	E
						Y								A	F
	H	E	P	A	R	I	N							L	O
						G	L	A	S	C	O	W			T
						E									A
D	E	C	O	R	T	I	C	A	T	E					X
	E				H			L							I
	G				I										M
					R										E
					D										

an identical piece. Initially, the player guesses the location of the match; then later as pieces are turned over and shown, the player remembers the location of the piece that makes a match. This game follows the same premise, but an additional step is added. The student turns over a mnemonic and must match the corresponding definition

TABLE 5.6   Crossword Clues

Across

18 Intervention of exhale while turning patient prevents this
20 Medication that decreases cerebral swelling
25 Causes pain along the spine when flexed if abnormal
31 Oral drug commonly used in the prevention of strokes
43 Causes an increase in intracranial pressure
46 Intravenous drug used with stroke patients to prevent more clots from forming
49 Scale used to assess eye opening, motor, and verbal responses
57 Abnormal posture in which arms are flexed and legs are extended

Down

11 A sign of a basilar skull fracture, _____ eyes
19 Type of testing contraindicated if intracranial pressure high, _____ tap
21 Type of suctioning contraindicated if skull fracture present
33 Cranial nerve tested by asking patient to smile, frown, and puff out cheeks
41 Antibiotic given to treat meningitis
58 Withhold caffeine prior
59 Cranial nerve that tests pupillary response

of the mnemonic. When uncovering and matching mnemonics to their definition, students must verbally discuss their meaning (see Figure 5.1). After completing all matches, the players with the most matches wins. This game could be played with several other different possibilities: medications (drug classes and their effects, drugs and their side effects, and drugs and their nursing implications); abbreviations and definitions; or names of diagnostic tests with nursing implications.

This is a quick game that reinforces memory of complex data. It can be used as a post–conference activity, as a study group aid, or as a class activity. The "drill" aspect of the activity enhances memory.

INFO LINKS

Another game, "Info Links," is based on the classic "Dominoes" game. Each player or team is dealt six info cards. Each card is divided in half horizontally and contains a different word or meaning on each side (see Figure 5.2). The meanings and words on each card are unrelated. A few info cards may say "wild" on one side, and these can be used as any meaning or word the player wants it to represent. The remaining cards are put in a pile in the center of the table face down. To begin the game, the first player turns over the top card, and it begins as in the traditional Domino game. In turn, players try to add to the chain. If

Abdominal Distention	9 S's Size Shape Surface Site Symptoms Softness Squeezability Spread Sensation	8 F's Fat Fluid Feces Flatus Fibroid Full bladder False pregnancy Fetus	Assessment of Cranial Nerve #3
Treatment of Sprain	Pain Assessment	Melanoma Characteristics	Assessment of Lump
PQRST Problem Pain Quality, Quantity Region, Radiation Signs, Symptoms Time of Onset	RICE Rest Ice Compress Elevate	PERRLA Pupils Equal Round Reactive Light Accommoda- tions	5 P's Pallor Pain Paresthesia Pulses Poikeothermy
ABCD Asymmetry of border Bleeding Color-blue black variegated Diameter ↑ 6 cm	Wound assessment	Circulation checks	REEDA Redness Edema Ecchymosis Discharge Approximation

FIGURE 5.1   Examples of cards for the ultimate memory game.

71

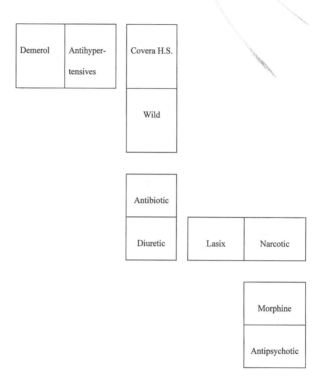

FIGURE 5.2   Info links.

they do not have an information card that "fits," they must draw from the pile, increasing the number of cards they hold. If players can add to the chain, they must explain why that information card fits and get agreement from all group members. The first person or team out of information cards wins. This game of Info Links is an excellent way to drill students on specific medications and their classifications, laboratory tests and nursing implications, or medical terminology and their definitions, to name a few.

NAME IT

This is a game that is based on the old television show, "Name That Tune." In preparation for the game, the professor or groups of students pick a concept, a historical nurse leader, a theorist, a complication, or other such entity. They create a list of "clues" that describe their concept or person, listing them from general to specific. A list of 6 to 10 clues per entity works well. Once a number of these has been created, student groups play the game (see Table 5.7 for an example). The "host" of the game, which could be the teacher or a student, along with two student groups play the game. A coin toss determines which group begins. A designated speaker from each group comes forward. The speaker from the group going first says, "My group can 'name it' in five clues," the other group's speaker can then say, "My group can 'name it' in four clues." This back-and-forth challenge continues until one group's speaker declines the challenge and says, "name it." The host then gives the other team the appropriate number of clues. They have 60 seconds to discuss the answer among themselves before the host asks the group's speaker to "name it." If they answer correctly, they get a point. If they answer incorrectly, the other team gets a chance to answer. If they answer correctly, they get the point. If they also miss, the host reads the remaining clues, and the first team to respond correctly gets the point. After each point is scored, a class discussion evolves about the entity being described. The team with the most points wins.

This is an excellent way for students to prepare for an examination or practice their skills of memory and identification.

WHAT'S THAT INTERVENTION?

This game is based on the television show, "Family Feud." Teams of four to six students play the game, two teams at a time. A student or the professor serves as the host and asks the questions. Any student can serve as the one who uncovers the answers as they are discovered. Before the game, the professor or student groups develop several nursing situations that require numerous interventions (see Table 5.8) and using an overhead transparency record the interventions and then cover the list so it is not visible to the players. Teams form a row on opposites sides of the host. One at a time, members come forward to represent their team. The host reads the scenario, and the first member who rings the bell sitting on the table in front of the host is eligible to respond with one intervention. If he or she is correct, this person may either choose to have the team complete the intervention list or pass it to the other team to solve. If wrong, the other team gets a chance. The host then asks each member of the team that is answering, in turn, to give an appropriate intervention. If it is on the list, it is uncovered, and the next member gets a turn. If the team gets three "strikes" or incorrect responses before uncovering all of the answers, the other team gets to collaborate and decide jointly on one intervention thought to be on the list. If this team chooses one on the list, these

TABLE 5.7   Example of "Name It" Clues

Placenta Previa

1. Vaginal bleeding is a symptom.
2. A complication of pregnancy.
3. It occurs during the third trimester.
4. It may require a cesarean section.
5. The bleeding is painless and bright red.
6. It can be partial, complete, or low lying.

Florence Nightingale

1. A historical nurse leader.
2. Felt nursing education should occur in a university setting.
3. Responsible for the first attempts at nursing research.
4. Nursed soldiers in the Crimean War.
5. Stressed cleanliness and environmental conditions in nursing.
6. Lady with the lamp.

group members can steal the total points for that scenario. Teams accumulate points based on the number of interventions they uncover. After three scenarios, the team with the most points wins. After each scenario, the instructor leads a class discussion on what interventions are appropriate, their rationale, and potential complications.

This game is also an excellent preparation for course examinations, NCLEX, or just review. It could be used by staff development or nursing supervisors as review for staff or preparation for certification examinations or hospital accreditation.

MEDICATION MADNESS

This game can be played by two groups of students in a classroom situation or by pairs of students in a clinical group. The faculty member puts the names of numerous medications on 3- x 5-inch cards and places them in a small paper or cloth bag. Posted on the board or on an overhead, the instructor lists the things students need to remember about medications, such as classification, normal dosage and route, physiological action, side effects, and nursing implications. One team or pair draws a card. They read the name of the medication and give an answer to one of the categories listed on the overhead or board. If they cannot come up with an answer, the other team or pair gets the chance to respond. The faculty member writes his or her answer next to the appropriate item on the list and asks the rest of the class to respond to its correctness. If it is correct, the other team or pair gives the answer to another item on the list. Discussion follows. This continues

TABLE 5.8   Examples of "What's That Intervention?" Situation

Situation: Jill Southern is 2 days postop from an abdominal hysterectomy. She is complaining of chills, is perspiring profusely, and says she feels "awful." In checking her dressing you note redness, edema, and small amounts of yellow purulent discharge. What do you do?

1. Take vitals—especially temperature
2. Call doctor
3. Change clothes
4. Keep culture of drainage for lab
5. Change dressing
6. Offer fluids
7. Document findings
8. Check laboratory values (i.e., white blood cell count)

until all items asked for on the board or overhead are filled in. At this point, the medication is reviewed by the class. A new card is drawn, and the process repeats itself. Each team or pair gets one point for every correct reply. The winner is the team or pair with the highest number of points.

This activity is an excellent way to review pertinent medications related to content area in the classroom or clinical unit. It stimulates discussion related to nursing implications and allows students to create and visually view important aspects necessary to know about specific medications. This enhances memory as students are active in the process of learning.

NURSE OF THE YEAR

"Nurse of the Year" is a great game to play with a few students. It is a good post–conference activity and can be designed in a variety of ways to elicit the content learning and thinking skills desired. In a small group, students play the game as the instructor serves as moderator and judge. The object of the game is to move a player piece from "Novice Nurse" to "Nurse of the Year." Players, in turn, roll a die and move the corresponding number of spaces on the gameboard. As players land on a space they must draw the designated card and answer the question correctly in order to remain on that space. An incorrect answer requires them to return to their prior location on the board. A few spaces do not require the student to answer a question. The instructor leads the discussion of each question, adds pertinent information students neglect to mention, and clarifies or corrects incorrect responses. One game board can be used with different card sets to tailor the learning to the objectives set by the teacher (see Figure 5.3).

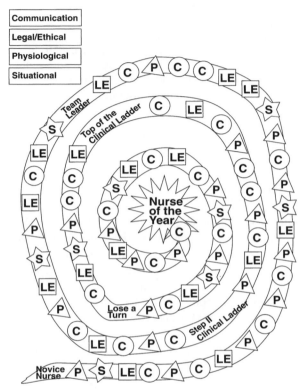

FIGURE 5.3   Nurse of the Year game board.

Table 5.9 shows examples of cards that might be used in game. In this example, the "S cards" reflect situations that might occur in the life of a registered nurse and direct the player to move ahead or back on the game board, or to miss a turn. "LE cards" reflect legal ethical dilemmas a nurse might experience, "C cards" situations that require communication skills, and "P cards" physiological concerns. Additional cards could be added to reflect management/leadership skills, nursing interventions, or other areas pertinent to student learning needs. The game could be played with more students by having pairs of students compete with other pairs. It can be adapted to serve the teaching needs of the faculty member and the learning needs of the student.

GAMING BENEFITS

There are multiple benefits to using games to teach content. First, students usually are anxious about tests. This anxiety often blocks their

TABLE 5.9   Examples of Cards for "Nurse of the Year" Game

LE Cards	Your 50-year-old client has been diagnosed with terminal cancer. The doctor tells you that the family does not want her to know the diagnosis. She is coherent and begins asking you questions about the diagnosis. What do you do?
	You witness a peer stealing codeine from the medicine cart. She tells you that she has migraines and cannot work without codeine. Her doctor refuses to give her enough codeine to allow her to work comfortably. She begs you not to turn her in and promises never to do it again. What do you do?
S Cards	• You were late to work; go back three spaces. • You forgot to update your cardiopulmonary resuscitation and liability insurance; go back five spaces. • You just presented a great staff development program; go to "Step 2 Clinical Ladder." • You got a merit raise; move forward two spaces.
P cards	A 56-year-old white man is postop for a carotid angiogram. His R femoral dressing is dry and intact and without swelling. R pedal pulse is strong and regular. As he is consuming his clear liquid diet, he dribbles the fluid out of his mouth, and you observe facial weakness. Anticipate what could be happening and other data you need to collect.
C Cards	You arrive at work and find you are the only RN for 30 postop clients. An LPN and aide are your only staff. Both are new employees and tell you they can handle only two patients each. Your supervisor tells you to "Get used to it—that's life!"
	It is 3 a.m., and your 10-hour postop nephrectomy client has a pulse of 120, blood pressure of 80/60, and a hemoglobin of 6. He is restless and complaining of severe back pain. You call the doctor, and she instructs you to "keep an eye on him and report back to me in the morning." How do you respond? What do you do?

ability to process and retain information. This method of test review is fun and reduces the anxiety and fear that often accompanies test taking. Also, games reduce the risk of failure as grades are usually not given. Learning in this way occurs more naturally in a nonthreatening environment. Second, games promote active, student-centered learning, allowing students to interact freely as they solve problems. This strategy causes students to focus on concrete tasks and forces them to become engaged in learning the material. Students are required to begin the review process early, especially when they are assigned the task of developing questions on all content covered in class. In addition, this task forces students to prioritize information, choosing only content that is most important for their questions. As a result, this content has the most potential for being covered on a test. Games provide an open-ended opportunity for students to clarify their ideas and ask questions. Discussion of the material during the game as questions are answered helps students process and remember the material. Listening to each other respond to the questions helps students validate their own formulated answers to the questions. It also clears up any misconceptions regarding the information. This active involvement, in which students formulate answers to questions and articulate their rationale to other team members, increases retention and understanding far more than passively receiving this through a test review lecture. Third, games provide immediate feedback. Students instantly hear the correct answer and can assess their own level of comprehension and consequently their need for further study. Fourth, games are highly motivating to students, whereas teacher-delivered factual material is often tedious and boring. Fifth, games promote cooperation and social learning—skills critical for team development.

In summary, this chapter has presented numerous ways to help students prepare for class as well as process information in class. Learning vital and essential knowledge is imperative for adequate analysis and reflection of the material. Study guides provide the vehicle for critical reading, whereas gaming structures provide practice in remembering and discovering their own learning strengths and limitations related to the material. This provides the framework for faculty to change their role from one of delivering information to one of facilitating active student learning.

CHAPTER 6

Writing as a Tool for Critical Thinking

Effective communication involves more than being able to express oneself verbally. Students need to be articulate in writing as well as in speaking. Writing allows students to formulate their own ideas and create a logical flow of thoughts. It also teaches them how to use words appropriately, build their vocabulary, and practice effective writing skills. When students are required to put their thoughts in writing, it forces them to reflect on their own ideas. It makes them consider their own value structures as well as analyze and critique the logic of their thinking processes. As nursing faculty, we must help students practice and perfect this essential communication skill. This chapter describes several techniques useful for implementing this learning outcome.

GROUP WRITING STRUCTURE: PASS THE WRITING

Traditional scholarly papers graded by faculty are but one way to help students perfect their writing skills. Group writing intensifies the learning as peers read and critique each other's writing. It provides the writer with suggestions to improve clarity, logic, and flow of ideas as well as gives additional supportive viewpoints or rebuttal. Oftentimes students feel less threatened by peer critique and supported as they work together to improve their individual skills. Faculty can transform traditional individual writing exercises into a group structure by first giving individual group members a topic or prompt to write about as a homework assignment or class activity. Each group could be given different topics to explore. On completion of the individual writing exercise, each group member passes his or her writing to another peer that

79

belongs to a different group and has responded to a different topic or prompt. The peer who receives the writing must respond with a written critique. Asking students to critique requires that the instructor first helps them learn how to do this skill effectively. Providing them with a written guide to record their perceptions helps demystify this new student role. The critique should include a variety of common categories based on actual writing skills and the writer's ideas and values (see Table 6.1). The original writing and critique is then returned to the original writer, who shares it with his or her group members (who have all written on the same topic). Group members combine, synthesize, and summarize their individual ideas on their assigned topic into one group paper through consensus. Each group then summarizes its main points in an overall class presentation and discussion. Both group and individual papers are then collected by the faculty member for grading or constructive criticism. This group writing format, Pass the Writing, provides a framework for faculty to use to implement group writing in their classes. It can be used in its totality, as described earlier, or adapted to the situation (see Table 6.2). The following are examples of topics or writing prompts that stimulate critical analysis related to nursing practice.

CLINICAL WRITING PROMPTS

Table 6.3 gives several examples of writing prompts that could be used as an ending to a clinical experience. Because most clinical groups consist of only 8 to 10 students and conferences are relatively short, the same writing prompt may be used for everyone. Students could pass their written work to the right or left, as they sit in a circle, for critiquing. These assignments could be given during pre–conference activity so students could reflect on them throughout the clinical experience or given as a post–conference activity. Instead of completing the entire process as explained in Table 6.2, the exercise could be adapted to save time by assigning pairs of students to correspond and critique each other's work via e-mail. Students learn how to record their ideas effectively, as well as how to critique others' writing abilities, ultimately learning or improving their own writing skills.

WRITING PROMPTS TO INCREASE INSIGHT AND PERSPECTIVE

An example of a way to challenge students who often have narrowly confined paradigms or lack of diversity in their ideas is for faculty to

TABLE 6.1   Peer Critique of Written Assignments

	NA	1	2	3	4
1. The values expressed are congruent with nurse practice act.					
2. Correct and logical interpretations exist throughout the paper.					
3. Sentence structure (complete sentences, no run-ons) is correct.					
4. Topic sentence exists for each paragraph.					
5. Correct grammar is used.					
6. Correct punctuation is used.					
7. There is a logical flow of ideas/ reasoning/assumptions.					
8. The paper has clarity—it is clear and makes sense.					
9. The summary clearly pulls together the total paper.					
10. The body of paper supports the topic sentence.					
11. The writer adequately completed the writing prompt.					

Comments—strengths and suggestions for improving the paper:

Critiquer's personal response to the essence of the paper:

Writer_____

Critiquer _____

Key: NA = not applicable; 1 = rarely; 2 = sometimes; 3 = usually; 4 = always.

require students to react to many different situations through writing (see Table 6.4). Through this type of writing exercise, students will begin to learn how their personal values and feelings related to differences might affect their nursing care or their working relationships. As student groups use the Pass the Writing structure (see Table 6.2), they will, it is hoped, develop insight into their own personal prejudices and broaden their thinking so that they can view the world from a variety of perspectives. This exercise could be used for small groups both in the classroom and clinical areas, and could be combined with another strategy, Academic Controversy (see Chapter 3), to add yet another dimension to the learning. Being exposed to opposing viewpoints and arguments helps students learn to appreciate perspectives different from their own.

TABLE 6.2   Group Writing Structure: Pass the Writing

1. Each group is given a different topic or prompt to write about.
2. Each group member individually completes the writing assignment.
3. Each member passes their individual writing to a peer in another group for critique.
4. Peers respond with a written critique based on specific criteria (see Table 6.1).
5. The critique is returned to the original writer.
6. Original group members meet and share their individual writing and its critique.
7. Members of each group combine everyone's ideas into a "group" writing on the assigned topic.
8. Groups report to the entire class and summarize main points.
9. Faculty grades or critiques the final writing products.

TABLE 6.3   Using Clinical-Writing Prompts

Writing Prompts

Write about your own development as a nurse after today's clinical experience.

1. Give five examples of your growth as a person and a professional.
2. What's the best thing that happened today, and why?
3. What's the worst thing that happened today, and how did you respond to it?
4. Give two new points you learned today that you will use in your future practice.
5. List two positive things the staff nurse you worked with did that you intend to emulate.
6. List two negative things the staff nurse you worked with did that you are certain you will never do.

TABLE 6.4   Using Writing Prompts to Increase Insight and Perspectives Related to Different Paradigms

Write your reaction to

1. Nurses who make errors in medications and procedures.
2. Male nurses who work in obstetrics.
3. Chemically dependent nurses who still practice.
4. People who live on welfare.
5. Parents who abuse their children.
6. Women who place their children for adoption.
7. Women who abuse drugs while pregnant.
8. Mentally ill practicing nurses.
9. Women who have abortions.
10. People with human immunodeficiency virus.
11. Homosexual patients or nurses.
12. Patients that are racist.
13. Nurses who fail state boards.

WRITING PROMPTS TO REACT TO READING ASSIGNMENTS

Often faculty ask students to read recent journal articles, research articles, or newspaper editorials. Traditionally, faculty have used the annotated bibliography format to assure that students have read material assigned. However, is it that we want to be sure the reading is read, or are we really wanting the student to understand, critique, and reflect on the author's work? The use of one or more writing prompts that focus on the critical thinking skills of analysis or developing insight into the author's assumptions can increase the student's depth of learning and make the article more meaningful for the student (see Table 6.5). These prompts require critical thinking rather than allow students merely to copy abstracts or findings.

Students learn to read critically and then express their analysis in written form as well as how to respond to another's analysis in an organized, thoughtful way. By using the Pass the Writing structure (see Table 6.2), students learn not only to critically think and critique, but also gain important knowledge from the information in the articles themselves. Stretching the student's thinking and requiring them actually to analyze and critique the author's assumptions results in a higher level of discussion when readings are covered in class, or when students are asked to complete a group problem-solving activity based on the readings.

USING GRAPHS AND INFORMATION AS THINKING PROMPTS

Students need to learn to interpret data from charts, graphs, and other visually displayed information as well as how to use written factual information to create these visual interpretations. Developing these skills is a part of learning to express data in a written form. One way to help students develop these skills is to give them examples of charts or graphs that present factual data and ask them in groups to write a narrative description interpreting the chart or graph example. They could also be given a narrative explanation of facts and asked to do the opposite, display the data visually in charts or graphs. Using the same template as in Pass the Writing (see Table 6.2), students could pass the graph/information. The skill of being able to explain charts or graphs as well as the ability to develop them are important to ensuring total understanding of the information. Also, being able to dialogue with others who have either interpreted the data differently or chosen

TABLE 6.5   Writing Prompts to Stimulate Critical Thinking in Relation to Assigned Articles/Readings

1. Summarize the reading in three sentences.
2. What are two major assumptions of the author?
3. After reading the article, what questions would you like to ask the author?
4. How could you use this information in your future nursing practice?
5. Did you agree with author or not, and why?
6. What additional ideas do you have that would support the author's viewpoint?
7. Write a rebuttal to the article/reading.
8. Explain the essence of the article to your classmate or a nursing colleague.

to display it in a different method help students realize the importance of accurately explaining or depicting data. Table 6.6 and Figures 6.1 and 6.2 give fictional examples of both processes; however, actual data could be obtained from sources, such as research articles or student surveys, if the instructor wishes. A variation of this activity could involve students in constructing, administering, and collating data, and depicting their results with both narrative and visual illustrations. This class project would give them practice in learning to write appropriate and clear questions as well as explain their results to others in clear, concise terms and visual depictions.

CASES AS WRITING PROMPTS FOR APPLICATION

Application is a skill faculty hopes that students will develop as a result of listening to lectures, reading textbook assignments and research articles, and practicing clinically. Sometimes this connection is not readily apparent to some students, who tend to view clinical situations and classroom experiences as separate entities. Faculty can use writing to strengthen this connection and reinforce their ability to apply theory and research to clinical practice. Table 6.7 gives an example of a case study in which students are asked to apply concepts related to theory. This could be implemented in the classroom using the group-writing structure, Pass the Writing (see Table 6.2). Faculty could develop case studies to illustrate a variety of concepts, such as chronic illness, family, developmental processes, teaching and learning, caring, or just one specific concept related to a nursing theorist (i.e., self-care, adaptation, conservation, etc.). Being able first to understand a concept and then actually use it in a case situation extends the student's learning and depth of comprehension. Application exercises etch concepts into the student's mind and enhance memory and future

TABLE 6.6   Examples of Narrative Information for Students to Chart or Graph

1. Healthy Home Care saw 873 clients last year. The ages of the clients range from 3 months to 96 years old. Twenty-four were 6 months of age or younger, 16 were 6 months to 18 months old, 8 were 2 years old, 47 were 53 years old, 62 were 81 years old, 76 were 64 years old, 121 were 73 years old, 61 were 60 years old, 96 were 77 years old, and 116 were 68 years old. Illustrate these data visually.
2. The following are the raw data from a survey done on 100 patients on a surgical unit related to pain relief. Illustrate these results.

	Always	Often	Sometimes	Rarely	Never
My nurse asked me to rate my pain on a scale of 0 to 10.	10	20	40	15	15
My nurse medicated me when my pain exceeded 5 on a scale of 0 to 10.	44	33	25	0	0
My nurse asked me if the medication worked after administering it.	31	14	20	25	10
My nurse prepared and administered my pain medications in a timely manner.	7	5	10	10	68

abilities to use the information. Again, writing prompts serve to expand the learning process by requiring students to think critically and relate concepts to real-life situations.

PRACTICE PROBLEMS AS WRITING PROMPTS

As nurses, students will be required to solve many complex problems involving clients or staff. The first step in solving a particular problem is to determine the cause. Table 6.8 lists several examples of problems students may encounter as practicing professional nurses. Faculty can use these problems as the basis for students to analyze individually and determine causes and plausible solutions in writing. After individually recording their thoughts, students can critique and respond to each others' responses; group and expand their ideas; discuss alternative causes and solutions; or, as a group, come to a consensus on the feasibility of the success of the chosen solution. Again, the group-writing structure, Pass the Writing (see Table 6.2), provides a framework for

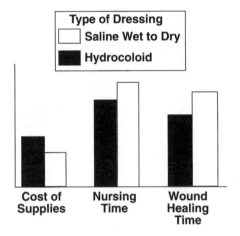

- Write a narrative explanation of this graph
- What other information do you need?
- What are your conclusions?

FIGURE 6.1 Examples of graphs using fictional data for students to explain.

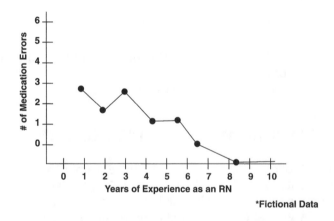

- Explain in writing your conclusions related to this graph.
- What other data do you need?

FIGURE 6.2 Examples of graphs using fictional data for students to explain.

TABLE 6.7   Case Study for Students to Apply a Principle/Theory To

Joe Sweet is a 78-year-old insulin-dependent diabetic. He lives alone with his dog, Barky—his only companion. His son, Sam, who lives nearby does not know what to do with him, as he eats only once a day and frequently has periods of hypoglycemia. Last week, Sam found Joe lying at the bottom of the stairs. His only injury appears to be a gash on his toe, where his toenail was ripped off. Sam has contacted a nursing home, but Joe refuses to leave his home because of Barky.

Complete one of the following:
1. Apply a nursing theorist of your choice to this situation.
2. Apply developmental theory to this situation.
3. Apply family theory to this situation.
4. Apply chronic illness theory to this situation.
5. Apply pathophysiology of diabetes to this situation.

TABLE 6.8   Common Problems Encountered by Practicing Professional Nurses

1. Staff nurses are refusing to care for clients getting abortions on an obstetrical unit in a major university hospital.
2. An AIDS patient is being ignored by the nursing staff as evidenced by the patient's report.
3. Staff nurses are restraining all confused elderly clients despite existing restraint policies.
4. A nurse observes her peer charting administration of gentamycin at a time other than when she did it, which will affect the drug blood level.
5. Staff nurses think an inadequate RN/patient ratio exists for safe care on their unit.
6. Dr. Doe demands that povidone-iodine be used to cleanse and heal a wound when recent research recommends a hydrocolloid dressing.

---

student groups to process and expand their ideas. Allowing students to first think about, then write about, and then discuss with others the common problems and frustrations faced by nursing professionals will give them practice in group problem solving.

BENEFITS

There are many benefits to using writing as an individual exercise, but group writing intensifies and multiplies the benefits. In the group-writing process, individual students must first formulate their own ideas and record them in a way so that others will understand their meaning. They must then critique the work of others, another aspect of critically thinking. Students who critique learn how to use specific criteria to evaluate written work as well as formulate their own evaluative ideas in written form. As a group, students formulate a final product that contains ideas from all members and expands the overall depth of thinking and number of thoughts that result in a better overall writing sample. Students learn to think about their own thinking (Paul, 1993) in relation to their own writing as well as the writing of others. They learn to summarize or explain information, organize their thoughts logically, and explain and illustrate data. The use of writing has many possibilities in all aspects of critical thinking and is vital to the overall development of the professional nurse. The group-writing structure, Pass the Writing (detailed in Table 6.2) provides a basis for writing activities. It is meant to serve as a template; however, faculty can adapt it to fit individual class time and learning objectives.

CHAPTER 7

Putting It All Together: Implementing Group-Learning Strategies

It is obvious from the literature that the use of group-learning strategies that allow students to be active and involved in the learning process help students learn more effectively than traditional methods. Yet these methods are not without problems for both faculty and student. In this new paradigm, the roles of both student and teacher change significantly, and it is inevitable that this drastic change in functioning will result in some frustration for both parties.

WHAT DO STUDENTS THINK?

If we are truly to evaluate this new paradigm, we need to address both the benefits and limitations of the strategies.

In analyzing our student evaluations from over 200 college students taking our classes that employed interactive methods, it was found that group strategies do have a multitude of student-recognized benefits. Only a few students noted specific frustrations as well. This analysis of student evaluations has helped us recognize limitations in our methods and design new approaches to overcome them.

Evaluation data were collected over an 18-month period through written and verbal comments. Students were asked to respond to open-ended questions, such as: "How do you feel about being in a class that uses group-learning strategies?" or "How do these strategies compare with the more traditional methods like lecture and discussion that you have experienced in other classes?" Also, specific strategies were listed, and students were asked to comment on each. In addition, the authors had focus groups or discussions with students as to the pros and cons and the effectiveness of these methods. Students were told at the beginning of the course that these were new and innovative strategies and that their opinions and reactions were very important to determine the usefulness of the strategies for student learning. Also, they were assured their reactions and perceptions would in no way affect their grade in the course.

Students' perceptions regarding our teaching methods fell into four positive and three negative themes. A few students reported negative feelings, but in most of the cases, students felt that the positive out-weighed the negative. Positive themes identified were the following:

1. *Increased understanding.* Students thought that the use of these group strategies helped them better understand the material. Many stated that they thought they had to become involved and could not just sit back and daydream. This increased their understanding of the material and helped them learn and retain the material. Active involve-ment was identified as a factor essential to greater understanding.

2. *Enhancement of social interaction.* Numerous students commented on the social aspects of group learning. They felt "connected" to their group members and learned how to communicate their thoughts and ideas more effectively to others. They also enjoyed meeting new peo-ple and finding new friends.

3. *Encouragement of self-reflection.* Students were able to recognize that they were being exposed to new and different ideas and values. Because of some of the activities and discussions, they were made to look at opposing viewpoints and really examine and question their own value systems. Although most did not change their own ideas, they did think they could better appreciate the positions of others with different opinions.

4. *Promotion of group interdependence and responsibility.* Students overwhelmingly commented on their feelings of responsibility to their group. They recognized the change from a competitive arena to one of cooperation. Individual competitiveness seemed to be replaced with group caring. Students began to care about how others did and wanted to help their group do well.

The three negative themes were the following:

1. *Time commitment.* Some students thought that they were required to spend too much time on preparation and class activities. They thought that this took time away from the teacher preparing them for the test and telling them what was important to remember.

2. *Resentment of peer learning.* A handful of students resented "teaching themselves" and learning from their classmates. They thought the teacher was not doing the job that he or she was being paid for, and that they should not have to pay to teach themselves.

3. *Ineffective groups.* A couple of students complained about their groups. They thought that they were put in a group that did not want to work or that had a few members who did not do their part. They thought it was unfair to them to have to work with people who could not function or chose not to function in the group-processing activities.

WHAT DO FACULTY THINK?

Students are not the only ones that cite negative consequences of group-learning strategies. Again, the literature overwhelmingly sings praises to the benefits of this new paradigm, and many faculty echo these praises; however, many other faculty members are finding it frustrating actually to implement these activities in their own classrooms. As human beings, we are all resistant to change, and many faculty members have a difficult time giving up the ways they are accustomed to teaching and the way they themselves were taught. Many feel awkward and uncomfortable at first or may have difficulty giving up the expert role and being the center of attention. Bevis (1989) relates that female nurse educators often have a difficult time relinquishing power as they have finally found a "voice" in our historically male-dominated culture and "are reluctant to give up this hard-won position." Also, many faculty members do not feel supported in trying new things and fear that their evaluation ratings will drop or that they will be criticized by administration or their colleagues for doing things differently from the norm. In addition, they fear students may react negatively when changes in teaching are implemented. Once they buy into the idea and actually implement the strategies, a whole new host of frustrations and questions emerge. How are groups formed? How are grades determined? How do I help groups interact socially as well as process tasks effectively? How can I assure that learning is actually occurring? They begin to face new problems that they are not used to and have no experience in solving. Often they revert back to their own comfort zone despite their beliefs that the new paradigm does result in a higher level of learning.

The purpose of this section of the book is to address these issues, problems, and frustrations that are faced by both faculty and students, as they teach and learn in this new educational paradigm. The following are common questions asked by faculty:

How Can I Incorporate These New Group-Learning Strategies Into My Present Lesson Plans?

Thinking about totally revamping and redoing lesson plans is overwhelming and is by no means necessary for the effective use of group-learning strategies. It is best to start slowly and become comfortable with the techniques before even thinking of using these methods extensively. Introduce the strategies one by one and begin implementing them in a class in which you feel very comfortable and have taught before. Use your old lesson plans, and add one new strategy at first. You might want to try a new strategy every week or every month to learn how to use them and then evaluate which strategies work best for you. If you are comfortable with the content, you will be better able to focus on the strategy and feel "safe" in experimenting with a new way of teaching familiar content. Do not feel you need to keep the students in the dark or make them think you are experienced in using these group methods. Share with them your reasons for trying them, and ask their assistance in helping you evaluate their effectiveness. Make them partners in your attempts to increase the effectiveness of their learning. If they feel a part of the plan, they are more apt to "buy into" a new way of thinking and learning that will decrease their resistance and frustration with changes in methodology.

Also, allow yourself to fail, but keep trying. Not every strategy works with every class. You may experience several less than successful attempts before you really feel great about the effectiveness of a strategy. Find a colleague or group of colleagues and support each other as you all try to be more innovative and creative in your teaching. Share your successes and failures, and talk about ways to help students learn. Nothing stimulates faculty more than feeling free to brainstorm and talk about teaching. Change is difficult for all of us, yet we all want the best for our students. We need to support each other as we all grow as educators. Supporting one another builds collegiality and makes all of us better teachers.

Can These Strategies Be Used in Large Lecture Classrooms?

It certainly is easier to manage smaller classes physically when group-learning techniques are used, but it is entirely possible to use them in larger classes. As the instructor, you must make the class seem smaller and more intimate. This can be done by walking around the class as you talk, calling students by name, and interspersing cooperative group strategies that do not require a lot of movement or disruption. For example, you might say, "find a partner, and using Think-Pair-Share (see Table 3.4), explain in your own words the concept I just discussed." After having a few pairs report their explanation, you can assess how well the concept is understood and determine if it needs more attention to assure student learning. Students are active and involved despite the large class size. They feel connected to the content and each other.

Another idea is to use short writing assignments dealing with application of and reflection on course concepts followed by small focused group discussion, to help students feel involved with the content as well as involved with their peers. In general, any strategy can be used in a large class so long as the teacher thinks it through and modifies the strategy to fit the physical boundaries of the classroom and the time elements that must be adhered to. It is the teaching strategy, not the class size, that seems to determine learning outcomes (Bonwell & Eison, 1991). Try a variety of methods, including both in and out of class activities, that require students to collaborate with one another and become active in the process of learning. Large classes do not have to dictate a "lecture-only" method of teaching.

How Can You Grade Group Work On An Individual Basis?

Grading is a concern for both students and faculty and remains a continual problem for those of us who rely heavily on group activities in our classes. Students feel a loss of control in relation to the grade they receive if the entire group receives the same grade for various amounts of work contributed. They resent people who do nothing and still get the same grade as those who really put in time on the project. Other more reserved and quiet students resent those who dominate, take over, and do things without consulting others. One way to factor in these unacceptable behaviors is to use peer evaluation as the basis for individual evaluation. Every student grades each of their group members on a variety of things including the quality and quantity of their work, their social skills and group processing, and other things inherent in group work (see Table 1.4 for an example). To prepare students for this evaluation, the professor must stress the importance of evaluating ones' peers. Supportive comments, as well as the need for improvement, must be included. Group members must also have time to discuss the evaluation form, ask questions, and feel well informed on the things they are expected to do as a group member. In this way, the peer evaluation will be fair and serve as a learning tool rather than a punitive activity. The faculty member averages the grades given to each individual student and that becomes part of that student's grade. In this way, students realize that if they do not function as an effective group member, their grade will be affected. Students believe that group grades are fairer when this peer evaluation is used. Also, faculty can see who is carrying the brunt of the work load in the group and who is slacking.

Faculty can also use a combination of group and individual grading in group activities. For example, if a group paper is submitted, students can be responsible for different parts of the paper. The faculty can grade each part individually and then the paper as a whole; each student would get a average of the two scores earned. Group presentations can be graded similarly, as a whole and individually for the part each student presents. In this way, collaboration and cooperation is essential, but people who do not do their part or do it in an inferior way are penalized in the grading process. Faculty who are concerned about the influence of groups' projects and papers inflating the individual student's grade require students to meet a minimum standard in all areas evaluated including individual objective testing. In this way, a student who falls below minimum standards on individual work could not pass a course because of the grade inflation from group grading.

What Do You Do About Absenteeism When Students Are Learning In Groups?

Absenteeism is a major problem and can hamper the effectiveness of group learning. To decrease it, faculty needs to make students want to come to class. This can be accomplished in a variety of ways, such as taking off points from the final grade for missing classes, giving pop quizzes that cannot be made up, or collecting homework and grading it based on a coin toss each class period. Students almost always respond and attend class if not doing so affects their grade negatively. Also, once the group bonds and they realize that they hurt their group if they are absent, they feel responsible to be there. Peer pressure can also be called into play when students miss class consistently. In classes where group learning is the norm, professors can required attendance and drop people from the class if they miss more than three classes, for example. They can also figure attendance into the course grade. These practices, too, will keep absenteeism to a minimum.

What Do I Do If The Students In The Group Do Not Work Well Together?

This whole idea of groups not working well together is a major problem for students and faculty alike. Although it is not an overwhelming problem in most groups, you can count on having at least one group per class that develops some problems getting along and completing the task at hand. This can be extremely disruptive to the faculty member and the students in the group. The best way to handle this problem is to try to keep it from happening in the first place. Building in the following concepts will help prevent these problems from occurring.

The *initial forming of groups* is an important task for the professor and should be done in a very deliberate and organized manner. In general, groups should consist of four to six members. In groups with less than four members, there are not enough ideas or opinions really to encourage critical thinking and problem solving. Groups of more than six are too difficult to control and work with. Too many ideas and opinions make coming to consensus or solving problems almost impossible. Heterogeneous groups are generally better in that there are more differences for students to experience. Groups should be heterogeneous for age, gender, race, ethnicity, academic abilities, special talents, and so on. In fact, it is often beneficial to administer survey questionnaires to determine learning style (Kolb, 1976) or personality characteristics (Myers & McCaulley, 1985) to assure even greater heterogeneity. The greater number of varying perspectives in a group makes more complete and effective team processing.

Team-building activities are also an important activity to prevent group problems. Although it may seem like a waste of class time to do this, it will prove to be a vital ingredient for an effective team. Teams that are enthusiastic and trust and respect each other will work better together and achieve greater academic success (Kagan, 1992). Group members need adequate time to get acquainted, develop identity as a team, learn to respect and value their differences, and feel a team bond. There are numerous things that can be done to help teams develop and feel a commitment to one another. One such activity that encourages members getting to know one another is "Guess the Fib" (Kagan, 1992). In this activity, each group member comes up with two true unbelievable facts about themselves and one believable fact that is not true. In turn, students state the three facts about themselves, and teammates guess which one is false. This activity helps students become better acquainted. To create a sense of team identity, teams might come up with a team name. There are also many team-building exercises available for building respect for one another and for appreciating group differences, another needed element to assure group-processing effectiveness. "Bafa Bafa" (Hummel & Peters, 1994) is a game that can be played to help students see and respect different cultural values. Students are assigned to two fictional cultures. After learning the norms and values of their culture, they interact with the other group and try to figure out the norms of each other's culture. It is most effective in teaching differences for student nurses. Such activities as "Survival in the Desert" and "You Have to Have a Heart" are examples of two other structures that can be used to encourage respect for differences (Kagan, 1992), although many more are available in recent literature. Taking the time for team building is essential for effective group functioning.

Teachers can also help students find reasons to value and respect others and even increase the self-esteem and participation of lower functioning or nonparticipating students by assigning competence to these low-status members. Cohen (1994) thinks that there is often a difference in the quality and level of participation of group members and that the more reserved and quiet student communicates a message of nonparticipation by his or her nonverbal and verbal actions, which further segregates them from those actively participating. Teachers can solve this dilemma in two distinct ways. First, by stressing that the group needs a variety of abilities to complete the task and that although no one student can possibly have all the necessary skills, everyone will have some of the skills necessary for success. Then, the teacher verbally acknowledges the specific skill the low-status student possesses. Perhaps they are an expert computer programmer or a talented artist. The low-status student feels more competent, and others see what the student can offer to the group task (Cohen, 1994). In this way, the group will function more effectively as all group members will be involved and feel valued and respected.

Group rules and roles need to be established immediately after group formation. These can be assigned by the professor, determined by a group decision, or be a combination of both teacher and group developed. Rules might include a variety of things that must be adhered to by all group members. Rules might include the procedure that must be followed if a group decides to eliminate someone from their group for not contributing or being disruptive, and the consequences of not following the rules. Rules should be stated positively, be realistic, be easily understood, and few in number. (See Table 7.1 for an example of common rules.) The use of assigned roles may also be used. The roles are usually rotated so each member gets an opportunity to function in all roles. Typical roles would include leader or task master, recorder, encourager, and substitute (see Table 7.2). Having rules and roles are essential structures that help teams function effectively.

Social skills development including group skills and communication is an important component to having effective group functioning. Often students do not know how to work in groups. They have been socialized to be competitive, not cooperative in their associations with

TABLE 7.1   Class Rules for Group Learning

1. All team members must participate and contribute their ideas and thoughts to the group.
2. Team members must work together and help each other. "One for all and all for one."
3. Team members must be prepared for every class by completing class assignments.
4. Team members must keep an open mind and listen to others' ideas and opinions.
5. Team members may criticize ideas but not people.
6. Team members may ask a group member to leave their group if they unanimously agree that that person is not abiding by the rules, they have informed the person that they are not meeting group expectations, and the entire team has had a conference with the instructor before the action.
7. Any member that has been asked to leave a group must either find another group to accept them; do the project individually, getting zero points for the peer evaluation and a maximum grade of C in the course; or drop the course.

peers. Before we can expect them to work as a team, we must teach them the skills they will need to carry out a cooperative group activity.

David and Roger Johnson have stressed the importance of groups defining and analyzing the roles each play (Kagan, 1992). They have identified "task roles" or the functions required in carrying out a group task. For a group to complete a task, it is essential that someone initiates the group activity and that group members give opinions, clarify information, elaborate on examples, and pull together their ideas. They also list "group-building and maintenance roles" or the functions required in strengthening and maintaining group life and activities. Behaviors of encouraging, mediating, relieving tension, and expressing group feelings are necessary functions that strengthen group cohesiveness. Other group maintenance roles that keep the group focused on the task are diagnosing, evaluating, choosing standards, and asking for group consensus. Additionally, they have identified nine types of nonfunctional behavior that do not help and can often hinder the group and the work the group is trying to accomplish. Such behavior is blocking, withdrawing, being aggressive, and seeking sympathy. If groups are given this information and are aware of some of the principles of group dynamics, they can better identify and analyze the dynamics of their own group—hence, begin to have the knowledge to solve those problems or stop the ineffective behaviors before they cause a group problem. Using mandatory individual and group evaluations help students see how both they and their group members are functioning and can be used as the basis for group discussion of the

TABLE 7.2   Typical Group Roles

Team leader	Supervises team, gets group working, and assures that all participate; resolves conflicts (with help of other team members)
Recorder	Takes minutes; keeps records of all material, assignments, finished work, etc.; records members' absences; informs absent students of group activities
Task master	Keeps the team working toward the task at hand; intervenes if group gets off task and redirects their efforts
Substitute	Takes the role of any member absent

group's effectiveness (see Table 7.3 for an example of such an evaluation form).

Other ways to help students learn how to function in a group could include the use of a "Group Grumbles Box." At the beginning of the first class, the teacher describes the use of the "Group Grumbles Box." It is a small covered closed box that sits outside the teacher's office. Any student can submit a group problem to the box if they would like help in solving it. No names or information is to be used that will identify the group or the person causing the problem. Each week the faculty checks the box, and for the first few minutes of class that day, a total class discussion evolves regarding how one should go about solving the problem at hand. If no problems are submitted, the teacher discusses a common problem, such as a group member who always has an excuse why he or she did not do the assigned part of the group project or a person who always insists things be done his or her way. These discussions give students experience in solving problems and give them concrete solutions to use if such a problem occurs in their group. It also makes everyone wonder which group or person submitted this problem and to whom it is referring, so if an individual thinks he or she may be the person being discussed, behavior may change before it causes a group problem. Students never know if the problem being discussed is one submitted by a peer or if it is teacher generated.

There are also several activities that groups can engage in to help them practice consensus building (see Table 7.4). One such activity is "You Have to Have a Heart" (Kagan, 1992). In this activity individuals first, and then in teams, prioritize from 1 to 5 who of the five fictional characters should qualify for an artificial heart to save their life. As the teams try to come to consensus, they learn how to communicate their values and opinions and respect the differences of others. Yet, in the end, they must negotiate and come to a consensus as a group.

TABLE 7.3 Evaluation of Group Processing

	Never	Sometimes	Usually	Always

Self-Evaluation

I contributed my ideas freely.

I listened objectively to others' ideas.

I encouraged others to participate.

I was respectful of others.

I paid attention and stayed focused
on the task.

I avoided behaviors of blaming, arguing,
expressing personal feelings, clowning,
daydreaming, and other nonfunctional
behaviors.

When conflict occurred in the group,
I tried to mediate.

When conflict occurred, I helped the group
analyze the source of the difficulty and
what steps to take next.

When decisions were near, I asked for
group consensus.

Comments:

Evaluation of My Group

We worked well together and avoided
behaviors of blaming, arguing, expressing
personal feelings, clowning, daydreaming,
and other nonfunctional behaviors.

We stayed on task.

We respected and listened to each other.

We encouraged and supported each other.

When conflict occurred, we effectively
analyzed the difficulty and proceeded
with a plan to solve the conflict.

Group consensus occurred.

Decisions were evaluated and measured
against our group goals.

Comments:

TABLE 7.4   Rules for Making Decisions by Group Consensus

1. Group members will listen, with an open mind and without interrupting, while all members express their thoughts, ideas, and opinions.
2. Group members will not argue but will discuss differences of opinion.
3. Group members will remain open to modifying their own opinions as needed.
4. Group members will seek to gain at least some agreement of all group members.
5. Group members will not vote, bargain, or trade to reach a decision.
6. Group members will understand that reaching consensus will be time-consuming but will result in all members feeling ownership of the final decision, which will increase its chance of success.

Other activities promote effective communication skills and allow students to practice these skills. In the activity "Island Maps" (Johnson, 1996) a deck of 30 cards is dealt among the group members face down. Each card in the set has an island shape drawn on it. There are matches for all but one island shape, and some islands have more than one match. The group must determine which card in the set is a single island. The rules state that the players can look at only the cards dealt to them, that they may not trade cards, they may not draw pictures or diagrams of the maps, they must keep their own discard piles, and they communicate according to established group rules. This activity requires the group to talk about the island shapes to complete the task of finding the single island card. The group that correctly identifies the single island card wins the game. It is a wonderful way for students to practice being specific and concise in their communication. These are skills necessary for effective group functioning.

If group problems occur despite efforts to avoid them, it is the teacher's responsibility to first diagnose the problem and then try to help students solve it. Often students need help in figuring out what the actual problem is, as they tend to focus on the symptoms of the problem rather than the cause. If it is the teacher that determines a problem exists, it is her or his responsibility to alert the group to the concerns and together try to diagnose the cause of the problem to solve it. If student groups are required to keep group minutes, they can serve as a valuable tool to help diagnose problems and their cause. Minutes should include members present, times and places of meetings, group role assignment if they are being used, and assignments and due dates agreed on by the members. By reviewing minutes, faculty can help students pinpoint problem causes in some cases. The use of the peer evaluation (see Table 1.4) as an intermittent check for all team members as well as a final evaluation tool can be useful in helping group members realize how their behaviors are being perceived by others. Often this alone will result in individuals changing their behaviors and solving the problem themselves. The bottom line in solving group problems is honest and open communication. Because students may not feel comfortable doing this or may not have the skill to do so, the teacher may have to facilitate and role model the appropriate ways to handle group conflict and problems.

How Do You Know How Much Time To Give Students To Process The Problems In The Group-Learning Activities?

Determining time limits for group activities is one of the most difficult things to determine as there is no hard-and-fast rule. It is important to give students enough time to process adequately, yet not so much time that they have extra time to socialize and "goof off." Experience is probably the best way to get a handle on this problem. When you first begin using group strategies, monitor time with a watch. Walk around the room and see how groups are coming along, ask one person in the group to stand when the group has finished processing the task, or ask one person to go to the board and write their group's solution when the group is finished. Soon you will have a better idea how much time to allot. The use of "Numbered Heads" (Kagan, 1992) promotes listening and active involvement in the group processing and is very effective as a tool in implementing group work and keeping everyone actively involved in the task (see Figure 7.1). Every student in the group is assigned a number before the activity. After the activity has been processed by the group, the teacher calls a number, and the person with that number in each group stands and gives their group's solution or goes to the board and writes the solution. Because students never know which number will be called, they are more likely to listen and stay involved. If everyone remains involved, time is used wisely.

What If I Am Ostracized For Trying New Ways By Both Fellow Faculty And Administration? Is It Worth It?

Nothing is more deflating to one's ego than being excited about a new way to teach and being "put down" for rocking the steady boat of tradition. To succeed, you need support, and if it is not there, you must actively create it! Find a buddy and help each other as you both try to become better teachers. Meet frequently to share your successes and failures, help each other devise ways to use group-learning activities in your classes, develop a creative strategy and publish it—nothing gets you more respect than being published in a refereed journal! If the journal publishes it then you have validation that it was a good idea,

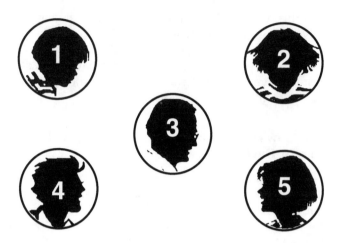

FIGURE 7.1   Numbered heads.

and you may find former skeptical colleagues asking more about your new methods. Perhaps volunteering to be on the faculty development committee will put you in a position to educate your faculty on this new education paradigm. You can encourage them to attend education conferences and read education journals, or you might circulate a new educational strategy from your favorite journal each month. If possible, encourage your department to hire a consultant to help everyone see the value in these group methods and help them integrate these strategies into your specific curriculum. Change is inevitable, and in time, we will all be expected to teach in accordance with this new paradigm, so let's embrace the change and not resist it!

How Do I Deal With Students Who Complain That They Are Teaching Themselves?

This is a common comment from students who are used to and accept traditional ways of learning. As with faculty, you must educate them as to the benefits of this new paradigm and win them over to at least giving the new way a chance. Tell them about what you are doing and why, and ask for their suggestions and evaluation of the strategies. Explain the new paradigm (see Table 1.1), and ask them to experiment with the new ways. Try to explain that you are trying to teach them how to think and problem solve, and reassure them they will learn and retain more if they apply information as is required in group-processing tasks. We need to help our students move from dualistic to multiplistic thinking (Perry, 1970). Thinking is a developmental process in which students make the transition from viewing the world in black and white to understanding that the world is really shades of gray.

What Do I Do If Student Groups Generate Unsatisfactory Or Incomplete Solutions?

The key to student group processing is preparation before class. If students do not have basic information about the concepts and content relevant to the group task, they cannot possibly be successful in completing it. Homework in the form of study guides (see Table 5.1) or open-ended reflective-writing prompts (see Tables 2.1 and 6.3–6.5) are necessary for students to complete before class and must reflect important and relevant information to be used in classroom activities. In this way, they have had the opportunity to read about and try to understand whatever the topic of the class is before class time and are better prepared to ask questions and apply facts to typical nursing situations and problems. Class time, while the teacher is present, is the time students should work on application of facts and information, as the teacher can serve as a resource person and facilitator. Using class time to repeat realms of facts that are in a book is a waste of the short time students have to interact with the teacher and their peers. Again, teaching is not telling. Once students realize that they cannot actively participate in the group activities if they are not prepared, they tend to come to class ready to work, and your problems are solved. One way to assure this preparation is to check study guides periodically or give students points for doing them. The use of a crossword puzzle, individually or as a group, could be used as a quick check to assure students are familiar with pertinent terms relevant to the class topic (see Tables 5.5–5.6). These methods help students become more self-disciplined in preparing and processing tasks in class. Also, an important teacher responsibility is to clarify information, correct misconceptions, and summarize the important points after the group activity. In this way, the teacher can assess the student's understanding and competence in this particular area. If it is apparent that students are not grasping the necessary knowledge, the teacher can try a new teaching strategy to illustrate the missing knowledge. All of these tips can help assure effective student task resolution.

I Don't Like The Feeling Of "No Control" I Feel When I Use These Methods, And I Don't Feel I Am Covering All Of The Material

First of all, realize that your feelings are normal ones. We all teach like we were taught, and we all resist change, especially if we feel we are doing a good job teaching in a traditional way. Before you will feel comfortable with the new methods, you must give them a chance. You need to accept the new paradigm and admit to yourself that teaching is not telling and that memorization of facts is not real learning. Try to integrate one group strategy into your lesson plan once a week and then increase it as you become more comfortable. In time, you will adjust to being more spontaneous and realize that the classroom is not out of control at all; rather, it is structured chaos, and you are the one who structured it! You will soon feel securer in not being able to answer every question they may have and feel good about showing them how to find the answers to their own questions in books, on the Internet, and by calling resource people. You are giving them the skills to solve their own problems, not only an answer to a question.

Covering content is another real worry for teachers. We feel obligated to tell students everything we know, and we still feel that the only way to teach is to tell. Again, we must change our assumptions about what teaching is and what learning is. We cover content in a new way, by asking students to read and prepare at home using study guides and then to apply the information in class group activities. One way to assure yourself that you are, in fact, covering the content is to use a variety of classroom assessment techniques (Cross & Angelo, 1988). Techniques like the "1-minute paper" can help you validate that you are, in fact, teaching students the content they need, just in a different and more effective way.

Yet another issue plagues all of us as nurse educators. What content should we teach? This question is more complex than is readily apparent. What knowledge is essential for students before asking them to think and process critically? As a profession, we have several levels of nurses, LPN, ADN, BSN, MSN, and PhD. The knowledge that each requires differs in both breadth and depth. It is this very issue that perplexes faculty. We, first as a profession and then as teachers for these various groups of students, need to determine appropriate learning outcomes for each of the levels. Once this is done, the subsequent problem of overwhelming students with impossible realms of information without helping them discriminate essential knowledge will be eased. However, it may be some time before the nursing profession details those delineations; with the knowledge and technology explosion facing society today, it is apt to remain a continued concern for all of us. In the meantime, you must decide for yourself what is most important and design study guides using focused questions that will help the student concentrate on the important facts.

SUMMARY

These are many of the questions faculty ask as they begin to implement these new ideas. It is hoped that these tips will ease your transition to group learning and ultimately enhance the learning potential of your students as well as stimulate you to continue to broaden your repertoire of teaching techniques.

References

Aronson, E., Blaney, C., Stephen, C., Sikes, J., & Snapp, M. (1978). *The jigsaw classroom.* Beverly Hills, CA: Sage.

Aumiller, L., & Rudloff, G. (1986). Decentralization reduces absenteeism. *Journal of Nursing Administration, 16,* 16–30.

Barr, R., & Tagg, J. (1995). From teaching to learning: A new paradigm for undergraduate education. *Change, 27,* 13–25.

Beitz, J. (1997). Concept mapping. Paper presented at the Nursing Education '97 Conference, Allegheny University, Philadelphia, PA.

Bevis, E. (1989). Clusters of influence for practical decision making about curriculum. In E. Bevis & J. Watson (Eds.), *Toward a caring curriculum: A new pedagogy for nursing* (pp. 107–152). New York: National League for Nursing.

Bigge, M. L. (1971). *Learning theories for teachers* (2nd ed.). New York: Harper & Row.

Bonwell, C., & Eison, J. (1991). Active learning: Creating excitement in the classroom (ASHE-ERIC Higher Education Report No. 1). Washington, DC: The George Washington University School of Education & Human Development.

Brookfield, S. (1989). *Developing critical thinkers: Challenging adults to explore alternative ways of thinking and acting.* San Francisco: Jossey–Bass.

Browne, M., & Keeley, S. (1990). *Asking the right questions.* Upper Saddle River, NJ: Prentice Hall.

Centre Productions. (1984). *Special care* (videorecording). Madison, WI: Wisconsin Educational Communications Board.

Cohen, E. (1994). *Status treatment for the classroom* (videotape manual). New York: Teachers College Press.

Cooper, J. L., & Mueck, R. (1990). Student involvement in learning: Cooperative learning and college instruction. *Journal on Excellence in College Teaching, 1,* 68–76.

Cooper, J., Prescott, S., Cook, L., Smith, L., Mueck, R., & Cuseo, J. (1990). *Cooperative learning and college instruction: Effective use of student learning teams.* Carson: California State University.

Cross, K., & Angelo, T. (1988). *Classroom assessment techniques: A handbook for faculty.* Ann Arbor, MI: National Center for Research to Improve Post Secondary Teaching and Learning.

Cuseo, J. (1992). Cooperative learning versus small group discussions and group projects: The critical differences. *Cooperative Learning in College Teaching, 2,* 5–6, 8.

Dailey, M. (1992). Developing case studies. *Nurse Educator, 17,* 8–10.

Dale, E. (1969). *Audiovisual methods in teaching* (3rd ed.). New York: Holt, Rinehart, & Winston.

Daley, B. (1996). Concept maps: Linking nursing theory to clinical nursing practice. *Journal of Continuing Education in Nursing, 27,* 17–27.

Dewey, J. (1944). *Democracy and education: An introduction to the philosophy of education.* New York: Macmillan.

DiFeliciantonio, T. (Producer and director). (1986). *Living with AIDS* (videorecording). Urbana, IL: Carle Medical Communications.

Ekwall, E. (1976). *Diagnosis and remediation of the disabled reader.* Boston: Allyn & Bacon.

Frederick, P. (1990). The power of the story and emotions in motivating students. Paper presented at the 10th Annual Lilly Conference on College Teaching, Oxford, OH.

Frierson, H. (1986). Two intervention methods: Effects on groups of predominantly Black nursing students' board scores. *Journal of Research & Development in Education, 19,* 18–23.

Galuska, L. (1995). Solve the puzzle of pediatric cardiopulmonary failure. *MCN, 20,* 334–336, 340.

Gandolfi, E., Tringali, S., & Cole, R. (producers), & Tringali, S. (director). (1985). *Don't cry for me* (videorecording). Brookline, MA: Umbrella Films.

Glendon, K., & Ulrich, D. (1992a). Using cooperative learning strategies. *Nurse Educator, 17,* 37–40.

Glendon, K., & Ulrich, D. (1992b). Using cooperative decision making strategies in nursing practice. *Nursing Administration Quarterly, 17,* 69–73.

Glendon, K., & Ulrich, D. (1995). Tic tac test ready. *Nurse Educator, 20,* 4–7.

Glendon, K., & Ulrich, D. (1997). Unfolding cases: An experiential learning model. *Nurse Educator, 22,* 15–18.

Goodsell, A., Maber, M., & Tinto, V. (1992). *Collaborative learning: A sourcebook for higher education.* National Center on Post Secondary Teaching, Learning, and Assessment. Pennsylvania State University.

Hummel, F., & Peters, D. (1994). Bafa Bafa: A cultural awareness game. *Nurse Educator, 19,* 8.

Ishikawa, K. (1982). *Guide to quality control.* White Plains, NY: Asian Productivity Organization, Kraus International Publications.

Johnson, B. (1996). *Island maps.* Proceedings of International Society for Exploring Teaching Alternative Conference. Columbus, OH.

Johnson, D., & Johnson, R. (1984). *Circles of learning: Cooperation in the classroom.* Alexandria, VA: Association for Supervision and Curriculum Development.

Johnson, D., & Johnson, R. (1989). *Cooperation and competition: Theory and research.* Edena, MN: Interaction Book Co.

Johnson, D., & Johnson, R. (1993, spring). What we know about cooperative learning at the college level. *Cooperative Learning: The Magazine for Cooperation in Higher Education, 13,* 17–18.

Johnson, D., Johnson, F., & Smith, K. (1991). *Active learning: Cooperation in the college classroom.* Edina, MN: Interaction Book Company.

Kagan, S. (1989/1990). The structural approach to cooperative learning. *Educational Leadership, 47,* 12–15.

Kagan, S. (1992). *Cooperative learning.* San Juan Capistrano, CA: Resources for Teachers.

Kolb, D. A. (1976). *Learning styles inventory technical manual.* Boston: McBer.

Lenaghan, N. (1996). Respiratory crossword puzzle. *Nurse Educator, 21,* 7–8, 14.

Lyman, F. (1987). Think-pair-share: An expanding teaching technique. *MAA-CIE Cooperative News, 1,* 1–2.

McKeachie, W. (1978). *Teaching tips: A guidebook for the beginning college teacher.* Lexington, MA: D. C. Heath & Co.

Myers, I., & McCaulley, M. (1985). *Manual, a guide to the development and use of the Myers-Briggs type indicator.* Palo Alto, CA: Consulting Psychologists Press.

Paul, R. (1993). *Critical thinking: How to prepare students for a rapidly changing world.* Santa Rosa, CA: Foundation for Critical Thinking.

Perry, W. G. (1970). *Forms of intellectual and ethical development in the college years.* New York: Holt, Rinehart & Winston.

Qin, Z., Johnson, D., & Johnson, R. (1995). Cooperative versus competitive efforts and problem solving. *Review of Educational Research, 65,* 129–143.

Sharan, S. (1980). Cooperative learning in small groups: Recent methods and effects on achievement, attitudes, and ethnic relations. *Review of Educational Research, 50,* 241–271.

Silberman, M. (1996). *Active learning: 101 strategies to teach any subject.* Boston: Allyn & Bacon.

Slavin, R. E. (1980). Cooperative learning. *Review of Educational Research, 50,* 315–342.

Slavin, R. E. (1983a). *Cooperative learning.* New York: Longman.

Slavin, R. E. (1983b). When does cooperative learning increase student achievement? *Psychological Bulletin, 94,* 429–445.

Ulrich, D., & Glendon, K. (1994). Fishbone strategy: A TQM strategy applied to nursing education. *Nurse Educator, 19,* 7–8.

Ulrich, D., & Glendon, K. (1995). Jigsaw: A critical thinking experience. *Nurse Educator, 20,* 6–7.

Ulrich, D., & Glendon, K. (1997). Let's play nurse. *Nurse Educator, 22,* 9–10.

Ulrich, D., Teets, J., & Quinn, C. (1994). Using video families to teach family functioning. *Journal of Nursing Education, 33,* 1–3.

Index

Page numbers in *italic* indicate figures. Page numbers followed by "t" indicate tables.

Springer Publishing Company

-FORTHCOMING-

Integrating Community Service Into Nursing Education
A Guide to Service - Learning

Patricia A. Bailey, EdD, RN, CS
Dona Rinaldi Carpenter, EdD, RN, CS
Patricia Harrington, EdD, RN, CS

This book focuses on the value of service-learning as an essential component of nursing education. Written by professors, it describes the role of faculty, students and community partnerships in the ongoing development of volunteer service projects. This field experience complements the classroom training, and bridges the gap between community and academic learning.

Designed as a guide to faculty, **Integrating Community Services into Nursing Education** stresses fundamental approaches. Chapter topics include an exploration of methods which teach students the reflective process, and an examination of the issues encountered in developing service-learning programs.

This book is an indispensable aid for nurse educators engaged in preparing students for their community involvement, and a helpful guide on preparing future health care practitioners for practice in community settings, as well.

> **Contents:** Preface • The Concept of Service Learning, *Dona Rinaldi Carpenter* • Integrating Service Learning into the Curriculum, *Patricia A. Harrington* • Critical Reflection, *Patricia A. Bailey* • The Promises and Problems of Service-Learning, *Dona Rinaldi Carpenter and Patricia A. Harrington* • Community Partnerships in Service-Learning, *Patricia A. Bailey, with personal stories by Peggy Begley, Janet Moskovitz, Tracy Lyn Svalina & Candal B. Sakevich*
>
> *1999   160pp (est.)   0-8261-1268-4   hardcover*

536 Broadway, New York, NY 10012-3955 • (212) 431-4370 • Fax (212) 941-7842

Springer Publishing Company

-FORCHOMING-

Teaching Nursing in the Era of Managed Care

Barbara Stevens Barnum, RN, PhD, FAAN

This book is designed to give nursing faculty a thorough understanding of managed care, in order to prepare their students for working in the managed care environment. It combines a clear and precise description of the many facets of managed care with cogent reflection on how managed care affects nursing faculty's practice, and the structure and function of schools of nursing. Graduate students in nursing education will also find this a valuable resource.

Contents:

- Acknowledgments
- Introduction
- The Managed Care Environment
- Problems and Promise in Managed Care
- Case Management
- Principles Underlying Managed Care
- The Ideology of Total Patient Care
- Resource-Driven Models
- Models in Nursing Management
- School and Societal Environments
- Nursing in the College or University
- The Nursing Program: Looking Inward
- The Education Process: How Do We Achieve It?

1999   168pp (est.)   0-8261-1254-4   hardcover

536 Broadway, New York, NY 10012-3955 • (212) 431-4370 • Fax (212) 941-7842

Springer Publishing Company

Evaluation and Testing in Nursing Education

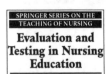

Marilyn H. Oermann, PhD, RN, FAAN

Kathleen B. Gaberson, PhD, RN

This comprehensive graduate level text is a valuable resource for nursing teachers, students, and health professionals involved in evaluating staff and developing protocols. The topics are organized into five broad areas: concepts of measurement, evaluation, and testing; test construction and analyzing; clinical and performance evaluation; interpreting and reporting test results; and evaluating educational programs.

Theoretical yet practical, **Evaluation and Testing in Nursing Education** features helpful models for improving the process, including numerous examples of test questions, and competency systems in health care settings.

Intended for use as a main text by graduate nursing students and as a handy reference for faculty, this book will also serve all health professionals concerned with efficient staff development.

Contents: Evaluation, Measurement, and Educational Process • Qualities of Effective Measurement Instruments • Planning for Classroom Testing • Objective Test Items: True-False, Matching, and Short Answer • Objective Test Items: Multiple-Choice and Multiple-Response • Essay Test Items and Evaluation of Written Assignments • Evaluation of Problem Solving, Decision Making, and Critical Thinking: Context-Dependent Item Sets and Other Evaluation Strategies • Assembling and Administrating Tests • Scoring and Analyzing Tests • Clinical Evaluation • Clinical Evaluation Methods • Social, Ethical, and Legal Issues • Interpreting Test Scores • Grading • Program Evaluation • Total Quality Management and Nursing Education

1998   336pp   0-8261-9950-X   hardcover

536 Broadway, New York, NY 10012-3955 • (212) 431-4370 • Fax (212) 941-7842

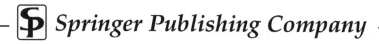

Springer Publishing Company

Telecommunications for Health Professionals

Providing Successful Distance Education and TeleHealth

Myrna L. Armstrong, EdD, RN, FAAN, Editor

"It is a book that describes how creative people, often taking a fresh approach, can get the best out of what modern distance communications technology has to offer."
—from the foreword by Susan M. Sparks, RN, PhD, FAAN and Michael J. Ackerman, PhD

This book is a guide to creating and managing programs in distance education and patient care, written by health care professionals with direct and extensive experience with these programs. Both the technical and human aspects of providing distance education and health care are addressed, along with practical information on how modern telecommunications technology can extend the skills of both the clinician and the educator.

Health care educators, administrators, and clinicians will find this book an invaluable resource to expanding their services beyond traditional geographical boundaries.

Partial Contents: Distance Education: What Was, What's Here, and Preparation for the Future, *M.L. Armstrong and K. Mahon* • Using Computer Technology to Provide Distance Education, *A.C. Hanson, C.J. Brigham and K.E. Hodson Carlton* • Support Services for Distance Education, *J. Repman* • Improving Telemedicine Consultation with TeleDoc, *C.S. Hickman and W.M. Dyer* • Practical Aspects of Telemedicine from the Users Perspectives, *M.K. Solowly Myers, et al.* • Ethics and Legal Perspectives for Distance Education and TeleHealth, *K.D. Menix* • Ethics and Legal Perspectives for Distance Education and TeleHealth, *K.D. Menix* • Public Policy Issues: Achieving Public Access to Technology at Reasonable Cost, *S. Cotton*

1998   352pp   0-8261-9840-6   hardcover

536 Broadway, New York, NY 10012-3955 • (212) 431-4370 • Fax (212) 941-7842

Springer Publishing Company

Fostering Learning in Small Groups
A Practical Guide

Jane Westberg, PhD
Hilliard Jason, MD, EdD

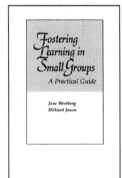

Drawing on years of experience, the authors address the questions that educators may have about small group teaching in the health sciences. The first half of the book focuses on practical strategies involved in planning and facilitating learning in small groups. The authors discuss the characteristics of effective groups and emphasize the importance of using a collaborative approach. The second half focuses on planning for and leading small groups that have specific purposes such as providing a forum for discussion and dialogue, teaching communication skills, and helping learners reflect on their patient care experiences, and more. The book's broad orientation and practical emphasis will be useful to all educators in health care.

Contents:
- Generic Concepts and Issues
- The Role of Small Groups in Health Professions Education
- Preparing for Leading Small Groups
- Preparing Yourself for Leading Groups
- Leadership Tasks and Strategies During Group Sessions
- Co-leading Small Groups
- Planning for and Leading Groups with Specific Tasks
- Facilitating Discussions and Dialogues
- Doing Problem-Based Learning
- Teaching Communication Skills
- Processing Patient/Client Care and Other Experiences
- Providing Support to Learners

1996   310pp   0-8261-9330-7   hardcover

536 Broadway, New York, NY 10012-3955 • (212) 431-4370 • Fax (212) 941-7842

Springer Publishing Company

The Mentor Connection in Nursing

Connie Vance, EdD, RN, FAAN
Roberta K. Olson, PhD, RN

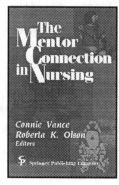

This volume explores the conceptual and practical aspects of mentorship and what it means in nursing. Over one-hundred nurses, including nurse leaders such as Joyce Fitzpatrick, Beverly Malone, and Marla Salmon contribute stories, essays, and personal reflections on mentorship. Their voices, in addition to the author's research, suggest that nurses are inventing a new, evolving, and very meaningful paradigm, which reaps mentorship's classic benefits:

- career success and advancement
- personal and professional satisfaction
- enhanced self-esteem and confidence
- preparation for leadership roles and succession
- strengthening of the profession

Mentoring is presented as an essential component of professional life, from student through high-level influential leader.

Partial Contents: Mentorship and Nursing • Mentoring for Career and Self-Development • Women Mentoring Women: Nurse to Nurse • Mentoring: A Song of Power, *Beverly Malone* • Mentorship: A Personal Perspective, *Marla E. Salmon* • On Mentoring: A Skeptic's View, *Barbara Stevens Barnum* • Tapping into Uncommon Wisdom through Mentorship, *JoEllen Koerner* • Mentoring: An Interactive Process, *Ruth Watson Lubic* • Full Circle: Peer Mentorship, *Caroline Erni and Susanne Greenblatt* • The Privilege and Responsibility of Mentoring, *Hattie Bessent* • Mentoring for International Educational Program Development, *Joyce J. Fitzpatrick*

1998   264pp   0-8261-1174-2   hardcover

536 Broadway, New York, NY 10012-3955 • (212) 431-4370 • Fax (212) 941-7842

⑤ *Springer Publishing Company*

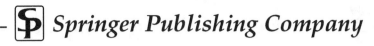

The Role of The Preceptor
A Guide for Nurse Educators and Clinicans

Jean Pieri Flynn, EdD, RN

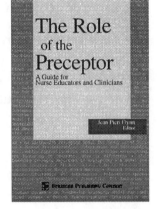

A practical "how to" guide for nursing faculty and administrators who want to set up preceptor programs, to guide student clinical experiences, or to help orient novice practitioners to the practice setting.

The heart of the book is the description of two model preceptor programs — one at a university, and one in a large, urban medical center — illustrating how these programs can and do work in real life.

Included are sample forms and procedures that can be adapted to your own institution's requirements.

Contents:

- Precepting, Not Mentoring or Teaching: Vive la Difference,
  B. Barnum

- Adult Learning Concepts Important to Precepting,
  M.J. Manley

- A Model Preceptor Program for Student Nurses,
  A. O'Mara

- An On-the-Job Preceptor Model for Newly Hired Nurses,
  J. Mackin and K. Studva

- Beyond Preceptorship: Internship and Externships,
  Fellowships / Apprenticeships and Mentorships,
  Anne Belcher

1997   152pp   0-8261-9460-5   hardcover

536 Broadway, New York, NY 10012-3955 • (212) 431-4370 • Fax (212) 941-7842